D0310893

# The Day Hospital

CHARLOTTE M. HAMILL is Associate Director of the Burke Rehabilitation Center, an affiliate hospital of Cornell University Medical College, where she is a research associate in the Department of Public Health. In addition, she serves as a program consultant to private foundations, governmental agencies, hospitals, long-term care facilities, and universities. She has developed and administered regional educational and training programs for allied health personnel in rehabilitation and long-term care. Her degrees include a B.A. from the College of New Rochelle, M.A. from Brown University, and M.S.S.W. from Columbia University. Coauthor of the book "Therapeutic Activities for the Handicapped Elderly" (Aspen, 1980), Ms. Hamill has also authored and coauthored various articles and papers in the fields of education and geriatrics.

# The Day Hospital
## Organization and Management

Charlotte M. Hamill, M.A., M.S.S.W., Editor

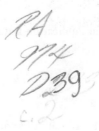

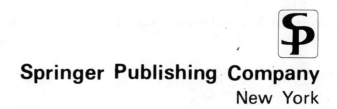

**Springer Publishing Company**
New York

Springer Publishing Company, Inc.
200 Park Avenue South
New York, New York 10003


81  82  83  84  85  /  10  9  8  7  6  5  4  3  2  1




**Library of Congress Cataloging in Publication Data**

Main entry under title:

The day hospital: organization and management.

     Bibliography: p.
     Includes index.
     1. Hospitals—Day care.  I.  Hamill, Charlotte M.
[DNLM:  1.  Day care—Handbooks.  2.  Hospital admin-
istration—Handbooks.  WX 29.1 D273]
RA974.D39     362.1'1          80-607802
ISBN 0-8261-3040-2
ISBN 0-8261-3041-0 (pbk.)




Printed in the United States of America

# *CONTENTS*

# PREFACE

This book addresses itself to those health care planners and administrators who are considering the possibility of establishing a day hospital program. For example:

>> *A private foundation in a small industrial community recently inherited a large sum of money with the stipulation that it be used for health care of the impaired elderly in that city. It currently operates a small nonprofit nursing home for elderly ladies, but has been advised by the state health department that its physical facilities are noncompliant with state codes. The nursing home care is considered to be excellent, and back-up medical services are provided by a nearby acute care hospital. The board of trustees has representation on the hospital board and on all of its key committees. An internationally renowned gerontologist was brought in by the foundation as a consultant to help them decide how to spend the recently acquired monies. The gerontologist advised them to begin with a survey of community health care needs for the elderly chronically ill and disabled. The major recommendation emanating from the survey was that the foundation establish a day hospital in cooperation with the acute care hospital and lease the recently vacated first floor wing of the hospital for that purpose. They now want to plan the day hospital program.*

>> *The administrator of two adjacent skilled nursing facilities and a retirement residence in a suburban area is concerned about the lack of treatment services for those nursing home candidates judged inadmissible to his institution. He would like to provide rehabilitation treatment by the day and enable them to remain in the community, with the knowledge that it is likely they will*

*qualify for admission in the future. He is also facing the problem of inadequate space for his inpatient physical therapy and occupational therapy programs, since treatment requests have increased in recent years. The retirement residents usually transfer to the nursing home when their self-care capacity makes that change necessary. He would like to offer the residents a daytime treatment program in an effort to delay their transfer from the retirement residence and enable them to remain in an independent living situation as long as possible. He needs to know whether a day hospital program operating in a building to be constructed adjacent to these facilities would be feasible.*

≫ *Health planners within an official health systems agency have surveyed one county within their region to determine its resources for the very large proportion of elderly, chronically ill, and disabled. It is a rural area, and their findings indicate a total lack of community-based programs equipped to provide comprehensive rehabilitation services on either an outpatient or daytime basis. As the official health planning agency, their commitment is to develop community-based alternatives to inappropriate institutionalization. They would like to determine the feasibility of establishing a day hospital to meet the identified needs.*

The situations just described are three actual samples of the hundreds of inquiries received from planners, administrators, health professionals, and trustees of health care facilities. The local scene and the principals vary, but the question remains the same—how can we start a day hospital?

When The Burke Rehabilitation Center Day Hospital began in March 1973, it was one of four research demonstrations funded by the Department of Health, Education, and Welfare.[1] Its major focus was the development of a comprehensive rehabilitation treatment service appropriate to the needs of physically impaired elderly patients who wanted to continue living in the community. Throughout the initial demonstration period and in the years since then, the need for specific information and guidelines has become increasingly apparent.

It is our hope that this handbook will provide the basic information and guidance needed by those who would like to initiate a day hospital program. Our aim has been to describe the process and the services in sufficient detail to give the potential sponsor an overview of what is involved. Any successful program undertaking, however, will need to be tailored to meet specific local needs and to qualify for current local reimbursement. Although the day hospital is relatively new to the United States, its individual rehabilitation service components are not unique. What appears to be uncommon is a sponsor's capacity and commitment to integrate those services into a program that maximizes their effectiveness within a therapeutic, patient-oriented environment.

The focus of our book is sharply defined and limited to the day hospital concept, which is sometimes referred to as adult day health services or the medical model of adult day care in the United States. It excludes adult day care programs that are primarily psychosocial in their services.[2] Psychosocial services are an integral part of the day hospital program, but its primary goal is comprehensive health care within a continuum of long-term care.

As reflected by the Table of Contents, this book represents a team effort with contributions by day hospital program and administrative staff. In addition, I would like to acknowledge the special contributions of Barbara Demmerle and Peggy Shannon to nursing guidelines and protocols. Invaluable assistance was provided in editing, typing, bibliography development and resource information by Joan Birnbaum, Ellen Blauner, Milica Dingwall, Edna Fernandez, Betty Lincoln, Betty Mercer, Mel Merchant and Helen Proctor. My deepest appreciation to them and to all the other dedicated day hospital staff who believed in the concept and made it a reality.

*NOTES*

1.  *The Day Hospital: An Alternative to Institutionalization.* Final Report to the Administration on Aging, Social and Rehabilitation Service, Department of Health, Education and Welfare. Grant No. 93-P-75203/2-03.
2.  *Adult Day Care Directory* available from Mrs. Edith Robins, Special Assistant for Adult Day Health Services, Division of Long Term Care, Health Care Financing Administration, Baltimore, MD 21207.

# CONTRIBUTORS

*Nancy Benes* has her B.S. from Colorado State University, where she also received her certificate in occupational therapy. She was the Coordinator of Therapeutic Activities within the Burke Day Hospital Occupational Therapy department from 1975 to 1979, when she became Supervisor of Occupational Therapy at Danbury Hospital in Connecticut.

*Barbara Berk* is a speech and language pathologist in the Greenwich, Connecticut, public schools. She received her M.A. in speech therapy from Columbia University and served as speech pathologist in the Burke Day Hospital for five years.

*Joan Birnbaum* is the Planned Giving Officer for Save the Children Federation, Inc. She received her B.A. in economics from Wellesley College and was an accountant with Price, Waterhouse and Company for four years. She served as Business Manager for Administrative Services at the Burke Day Hospital.

*Robert C. Oliver* is a clinical psychologist who earned his M.A. at New York University and has been Associate Professor of Psychology at Pace University, New York, since 1973. He served as codirector of the Burke Day Hospital research demonstration and of the DHEW Experiment and Demonstration for Day Care Services at the Burke Day Hospital.

*Maureen Ryan* received her M.S. as a Clinical Specialist in Psychiatric Nursing from Adelphi University. She was the Assistant Administrator and Coordinator of Clinical Services at the Burke Day Hospital for five years. In 1980 she became project director of the Westchester County Project on Access to Health Care for the Developmentally Disabled.

*Renee Schlesinger* received her B.S. and diploma in physical therapy from Simmons College. She established and directed the physical therapy department in the Burke Day Hospital for six years.

*Juliana Snyder* is a registered dietitian and nutritional consultant who received her B.S. degree in dietetics and institutional management from Ohio State University. She was the Nutrition Consultant to the Burke Day Hospital and serves as a consultant to many long-term care facilities.

*Joyce Vitale*, of the Burke Rehabilitation Center Speech Pathology Services, received her M.A. degree from Temple University. She established the speech pathology department in the Burke Day Hospital and directed it for five years.

ROBERT C. OLIVER

CHAPTER ONE

# The Day Hospital Concept

## DEFINITION

Farndale, in his report on the day hospital movement, notes that the term "day hospital" has a wide meaning.[1] Harris describes the day hospital as ". . . a place in which patients spend a substantial portion of their waking time under a therapeutic regime and from which they return to their own home or hostel at night."[2] The day hospital, as it has emerged in the United States, is a special type of outpatient setting. It operates on the professional level of a hospital, under the legal certification of the parent institution—usually a general hospital or rehabilitation hospital to which it is attached. It provides diagnostic and treatment services that do not require surgical intervention or inpatient care on a 24-hour basis. Its patients are usually brought to the facility in the morning; they spend approximately five to six hours in a program of treatment that is specially developed on the basis of their individual needs and then return to their homes.

The day hospital differs from the conventional outpatient setting or clinic in a number of ways. The range of therapeutic services is about the same as might be found in a comprehensive outpatient setting; the services themselves are, however, much more closely integrated, because they are part of a highly structured, comprehensive, multidisciplinary treatment/care plan that has been prepared on the basis of a very thorough assessment of the patients' health care needs. Rehabilitation services are emphasized, and management of the patient stresses his participation, as well as that of family members or others. Positive support for the emotional needs of the patient and family is provided as needed; purposeful activity is encouraged. Where possible, inpatient hospitalization is avoided, but it is made available when and as needed. The day hospital offers a setting in which the patient can be observed over a period of several hours as participation in the treatment program goes on. This observation provides a unique opportunity for evaluating how a patient cooperates in the treatment plan, what use is made of the therapeutic services, and the degree to which advances in activities of daily living can be sustained. It also offers an opportunity to involve the family members in the treatment and care of the patient, so that continuity of care can be maintained when the patient is away from the day hospital.

## HISTORICAL OVERVIEW OF DAY HOSPITALS

Day hospitals, according to Farndale, originated in Moscow in 1932.[3] Harris puts the original date as 1942, also in Russia.[4] The first day hospital in the English-speaking world was started in Montreal, Canada, as part of the Allen Memorial Institute, a psychiatric teaching hospital[5]; this was followed by a day hospital as part of the Montreal General Hospital, a large facility with a psychiatric department.[6] In the United States, the earliest day hospitals were also psychiatric and were founded at the Yale Psychiatric Clinic in 1948 and at the Menninger Clinic in Kansas in 1949. The Yale program included both a day and a night plan.[7]

The first day hospital in England started in London as an independent facility not connected with an existing hospital.[8] It grew out of the Social Psychotherapy Centre that began in London in 1946, came into the National Health Service in 1948, and moved to Marlborough Place in 1954 with considerably expanded services.[9]

In the period since then, the day hospital movement has grown apace, particularly in Great Britain where the growth has been almost phenomenal. There are well over 200 day hospitals caring primarily for geriatric patients who are both physically and mentally disabled. The development of the day hospital for geriatric patients is now a major part of the health care delivery system in the United Kingdom.[10] The first of the geriatric day hospitals evolved when "outpatients came to wards and rehabilitation departments of hospitals for the day, being taken home in the late afternoon."[11] The Cowley Road Hospital, Oxford, a part of the United Oxford Hospitals, was the site of the first purpose-built day hospital. Intended for the care of both the physically and the psychiatrically disabled, it opened in 1958, under the directorship of Dr. Lionel Cosin. Treatment emphasis was given to those in need of psychiatric care.[12] This hospital has served as a model for subsequent day hospitals that have begun to play such a significant part in health care in Great Britain. In his national survey of day hospitals, Brocklehurst found that consultant geriatricians placed most importance on the physical rehabilitation and physical maintenance of patients. In sharp contrast to this emphasis is that urged by Dr. Cosin, who pioneered in the concept of total patient care. He pointed out that in dealing with the patients who are served by a day hospital, it is not enough to deal with the medical problems; rather, he noted, the psychological and social problems are inextricably interwoven with the medical needs of the patient and must be considered in the treatment plan.[13]

## DAY HOSPITALS TODAY

A look at day hospitals in other countries shows that they are currently found here and there in Europe and in other parts of the world. A few countries, such as the USSR and Canada, have well-established day hospital programs for psychiatric patients. Day hospitals for physically impaired individuals exist in countries such as Israel, the Netherlands, Sweden, Denmark, and Australia. The day hospital is now a widely accepted part of the health care delivery system in the United Kingdom, and the geriatric day hospital, in particular, has become a bridge between the inpatient hospital and the community.

The partial hospitalization approach represented by the day hospital brings the resources of the traditional hospital facility to bear on the patient's problems, while, at the same time, avoiding the dependence and infantilization of the patient that is often associated with round-the-clock inpatient care. The day hospital can close a major gap in the continuum of treatment services—namely, comprehensive, integrated medical and psychosocial care without institutionalization. It helps the patient maintain contact with his personal physician. Actually, it enhances the relationship, because the personal physician is involved in the development and ratification of the individual health care plan developed in the day hospital.

The day hospital offers a new health care option in the United States for the chronically ill, physically disabled individual, regardless of age. The history of the psychiatric day hospital indicates that it is considered in the United States to be a viable, useful part of the delivery of psychiatric care. The day hospital serving individuals with physical illness, particularly the chronically ill, has the potential for becoming an equally viable option.

*NOTES*

1. Farndale, James, *The Day Hospital Movement in Great Britain* (New York: Pergamon Press, 1961).
2. Harris, Arthur, "Day Hospitals and Night Hospitals in Psychiatry," *The Lancet*, April 6, 1957.
3. Farndale, *The Day Hospital Movement in Great Britain.*
4. Harris, "Day Hospitals and Night Hospitals in Psychiatry."
5. Cameron, D. E., "The Day Hospital" in Bennett, A. E., E. A. Hargrove, and B. Engle, *The Practice of Psychiatry in General Hospitals* (Los Angeles, Calif.: University of California Press, 1956).
6. Harris, "Day Hospitals and Night Hospitals in Psychiatry."
7. Kramer, Bernard, *Day Hospitals: A Study of Partial Hospitalization in Psychiatry* (New York: Grune & Stratton, Publishers, 1962).
8. Harris, "Day Hospitals and Night Hospitals in Psychiatry."
9. Farndale, *The Day Hospital Movement in Great Britain.*
10. Brocklehurst, J. C., *The Geriatric Day Hospital* (London: King Edward's Hospital Fund, 1970).
11. Ibid.
12. Ibid.
13. Cosin, Lionel Z., "Rehabilitation of the Older Patient," *World Hospitals*, Vol. 9, October 1973.

## CHAPTER TWO

# Planning a Day Hospital

## SPONSORSHIP

The lack of an integrated system for the delivery of health and social services to the chronically ill, functionally impaired segment of our population is a result of the pluralistic approach to the delivery of those services. Health and social services—public and private—are delivered by specialized providers and tend to be organized as well as financed along categorical lines. Although this approach may increase the number of options in service delivery, it also increases fragmentation and inaccessibility for those individuals seeking treatment and care.

The decision to establish a day hospital program in a community is a commitment to increase the health care options and to make the integration of long-term care services on behalf of patients a reality. The sponsor may be a consortium of agencies, an official department of health or social services, a chronic disease or rehabilitation hospital, a rehabilitation center, or a skilled nursing facility. In some instances, it might be a community mental health center. Whatever the source of sponsorship, the rationale for establishing a day hospital program must be relevant to the existing continuum of care within that community. The sponsoring facility may provide all services directly, through referral, or in collaboration with other providers. If it is a governmental program administered from a central location in a state, it is possible that there will be a number of local sponsors with

policies and procedures formulated and regulated by the governmental agency. When the health care services to be delivered are an
integral part of the overall program of the sponsoring facility, it is
more likely that there will be continuity of care for the participants.
The availability of adequate back-up medical services, consultation,
and supportive services ensures the quality of the program and
broadens its scope. The sponsor assumes the ultimate responsibility
for the administration, coordination, and financial support of the
program, no matter what the structure of the program may be. There
may be contractual arrangements with other agencies within the
community network of social and health services, or the entire package of services may be delivered directly by the sponsoring facility.
The program goals must be compatible with the sponsor's overall
program goals, and it must have the financial capability of planning,
developing, and sustaining the contemplated program.

### PLANNING PROCESS

The planning process involves the following sequence of steps:

A.   survey of community needs and resources;
B.   analysis of survey and identification of unmet needs;
C.   setting of specific objectives related to unmet needs;
D.   development and implementation of a specific course of action;
E.   ongoing program evaluation.

The planning effort must be adequately staffed and have the
administrative endorsement of the governing body. If it is a cooperative
community-wide effort, a representative task force may be formed
for the initial survey; but the final decisions regarding the specific
program developed will be the responsibility of the sponsoring
agency's governing body.

The following is a description of each of the steps in the planning
process:

### A.   Survey of Community Needs and Resources

State, regional, and local planning agencies, such as health
systems agencies, area agency on aging, and health department, should
be consulted to find out whether any relevant studies have been made

of long-term care needs, to learn about their short-range and long-range plans, and to determine what steps must be taken to gain their official approval and cooperation. These agencies should be knowledgeable about existing regulations, the approval process, and reimbursement mechanisms. Regulatory mechanisms and policies are often restrictive in the scope of services that can be offered, making it important to be informed on such restrictions early in the planning process. Liaison needs to be established at federal, state, and regional levels for the purpose of information sharing and advocacy. The potential sponsor will want to make regulatory bodies aware of its interest in developing a day hospital program and should find out whether such a program is compatible with their current findings and plans. Since the planning process of the area agency on aging and the health systems agency call for participation by consumers, an effort should be made to have day hospital advocates serve on these planning bodies. Most planning agencies require extensive documentation of need in applications for new health care programs. Those requirements should be considered in the design of the assessment of community needs and resources.

For any health care program, the first step in the planning process is the assessment of community needs. If the geographical area to be served has already been established, then the assessment of need may be focused on what types of patients will be treated. Will they be physically impaired—psychiatrically impaired—developmentally disabled? What levels of functional impairment are to be treated? In certain situations, the patient population will be predetermined by the established purpose of the parent agency. If the sponsor is the Multiple Sclerosis Society, for example, the patient population would probably be limited to that as a primary diagnosis. Their assessment of need would focus on determining whether there are enough potential registrants in the community and what their specific treatment needs are. If these needs are more psychosocial than physical, the program contents and staffing will be designed accordingly.

A sponsoring agency that has established physical facilities, staff, and a specific program commitment may be interested in expanding utilization through the addition of a day hospital program within those facilities. Its approach to a community needs assessment will differ from that of a sponsor who is planning to construct a day hospital with no prior program commitments. No matter what the circumstances, day hospital planners must be knowledgeable about long-term care needs and resources of their particular community. If that knowledge has been acquired over a long period of time wherein they have been delivering health care services to the same community, their knowledge base will be more substantial; if this is not the case, then it will be important to seek all available sources of information as a basis for planning.

Many agencies serving the elderly and chronically ill will have a wealth of information to share regarding the service needs of the potential day hospital population. They may not have the needs carefully documented because most agencies, with the possible exception of an information and referral agency, cannot afford the staff time required to maintain such records. However, in-depth structured interviews with key personnel will reveal the gaps that are readily identifiable in their day-to-day operations. Hospital discharge planners, home health agency staff, private physicians, nursing home admissions staff, public assistance agency caseworkers, senior and nutrition center directors will all have firsthand knowledge of service needs. Consultation should also be arranged with Social Security Administration, departments of mental health, health maintenance organizations, housing authorities, offices for services to the disabled, transportation authorities, community action, and consumer groups. They should be interviewed in order to learn community needs as perceived by them and to seek their advice and reactions to the proposed day hospital.

The information-gathering process is time consuming but vital, and if the day hospital sponsoring agency is already known to these community resources for its commitment to quality care for the chronically ill in other programs, the task of gaining their cooperation and interest will be simplified. In the process of seeking data, it will be necessary to define broadly the purpose and treatment program tentatively envisioned for the day hospital in order to elicit information regarding potential duplication of existing services and to allay fears of professional competition. A home health agency that is underutilized, for example, would have a legitimate concern if the day hospital is going to offer the same services at a central location as the agency currently offers and if its patients are going to be eligible for these services. These information-sharing interviews also provide the opportunity to explore potential cooperative arrangements in the delivery of certain services that may not be available at the proposed day hospital. An area office on aging nutrition center may be in a position to deliver meals to the day hospital, a local rehabilitation facility may be willing to provide a part-time physical therapist on a contractual basis, and so forth.

The data gathered should indicate what long-term care treatment needs are not being met in the community and to what extent those needs have been identified and quantified. Quantification of need is the most difficult dimension to obtain but most important to program planning. If money and time permit, a formalized community needs study may be achieved. An example of such a study is the *Study of the Needs of the Elderly and of Resources Available to Meet Need*, undertaken by the Division of Research, Planning, and Program Development of the Department of Health and Social Development in the Province of Manitoba, Canada and published in 1973. (A diagram of the Manitoba study design appears in Appendix A.)

### B.  Analysis of Survey and Identification of Unmet Needs

Having surveyed the existing needs and resources, the next step is to analyze that information and identify the unmet needs that pertain to the day hospital being contemplated. If the findings indicate that there is a large population of functionally impaired adults who require rehabilitation treatment in a daytime program, but transportation is not available in one part of the region, it is reasonable to assume that the program cannot serve that segment of the population unless a transportation capability is developed. And unless there is a simple solution to that lack of transportation, it would be impractical for the day hospital to attempt serving that group. If the survey reveals a paucity of information about unmet health needs in one part of the community, then one of the program objectives developed may be a special community outreach effort. All information needs to be analyzed from the particular viewpoint of the sponsor and in light of the sponsoring agency's own commitments and priorities.

In the identification of unmet needs it will be necessary to consider whether the role of any current agencies can be expanded to meet those needs, or whether it would be more effective and appropriate for the proposed day hospital program to deliver those services. Interagency arrangements, shared facilities, shared services, and other alternatives should be given due consideration.

### C.  Setting of Specific Objectives Related to Unmet Needs and Available Resources

Setting specific objectives to meet the needs of an identified patient population for whom the day hospital service will be designed will determine the specific services to be offered. In the event that it is found that the greatest unmet need is rehabilitation for stroke patients and the goal is established to meet that need, a comprehensive rehabilitation program would be in order. However, if the findings also indicate that reimbursement for stroke rehabilitation is not available on an outpatient basis for certain services—such as nursing and social work—those factors must be considered in the program design and in any plans for private funding.

The utilization of other support services should be considered in this planning stage and written agreements formulated with cooperating agencies. The services of a nutritionist from a local health department or of a consultant from a local health care facility, or other such assistance, may be offered in early discussions. Clarification and commitment in the formulation of any agreements will prove to be useful and time-saving.

### D.   Development and Implementation of a Specific Course of Action

The final development and implementation of the day hospital program will build upon earlier planning efforts, particularly the liaisons established at federal, state, and local levels. The process will vary from community to community, but it is likely that it will require a number of assurances. The sponsoring agency should have a philosophical commitment to the day hospital concept and a financial contingency capability of maintaining the program service core in the event that reimbursement policies are suddenly reversed by third-party payers. Established working relationships with other community agencies and facilities, as well as demonstrated standards of quality care in its existing programs, are factors that will contribute to official approval and community acceptance of the proposed program. The official recognition and approval of the program will be required for purposes of rate-setting and reimbursement by governmental and private health insurance carriers. Since individual interpretations of regulations and policies will vary, it is advisable to get such interpretations in writing, especially if they relate to reimbursement and legal sanction of the program.

Day hospital planners should not underestimate the amount of time that will be needed for continuing interpretation of the program. An adequate description of the program objectives and services in relation to community need will usually evoke enthusiastic endorsement of the concept. But, unfortunately, such program innovations tend to be well in advance of reimbursement mechanisms. Consequently, the day hospital advocates will need to establish an ongoing campaign of documentation and interpretation of the need to state legislators, local officials, other advocacy groups, and congressional representatives.

In view of restrictive policies and limited funding, the initial program objectives may be more limited than the established goals. However, demonstrated success in quality patient care combined with marketing efforts should lead to gradual expansion. In those states where Medicaid has included the day hospital in its State Plan for Title XIX funds, for example, a day hospital program may initially serve only Medicaid clients. However, its visibility and success may eventually encourage the participation of self-pay patients and the support of select insurance companies. Planning requires not only goal identification, definition of specific programs, designation of the target population, and a description of implementation, including funding, but also a method of evaluation or monitoring.

### E.   Ongoing Program Evaluation

Program monitoring and evaluation should be a continuing process for the purpose of determining whether the program goals are being met and whether the requirements of regulatory agencies have been fulfilled. Program administrators are responsible for compliance with local, state, and federal regulations pertaining to reporting requirements. If the data generated for those purposes can serve a dual function of internal monitoring, this represents a saving in cost and in avoiding duplication of effort. The patient assessment process, as described elsewhere, serves as a built-in tool for program evaluation for staff because it makes possible the determination and measurement of goal achievement on an individual basis for those patients the day hospital was designed to serve.

### FACILITY PLANNING

The physical facilities and site for the day hospital must first meet the standards of any regulatory agencies having legal jurisdiction over the program. Ordinarily there will be the state and local health and fire departments, whose life safety, sanitation, and building codes must be met. If the sponsoring agency is part of a large organization that is subject to accreditation standards, these must also be taken into consideration. Those planning the conversion into a day hospital of a facility that was not designed to accommodate disabled individuals will find that there is literature available on making buildings accessible to the disabled from the National Center for Barrier-Free Environments in Washington, D.C.

The location of the day hospital should be as convenient as possible to available transportation. If it is part of a housing or retirement complex where individuals will not need to be transported from the outside community, the location should be convenient to the source of food service and to administrative offices. Access to and from adequate parking facilities is also important for the benefit of family and friends who may assist in transporting participants to the program.

Unfortunately, it is unusual for a day hospital to have the options of selecting a location and designing and constructing a purpose-built facility. It is more often the case that a program will be located in a physical area that is being reassigned or even shared. The problems of meeting overhead and maintenance costs or of too little space to meet all the service demands are common. Although it can be inconvenient and places demands upon the flexibility of staff, it is very helpful in the early stages of development to begin small and to avoid excessive overhead costs. The latter will increase the fees charged to patients and may serve as a deterrent to the program's growth and fiscal feasibility. It is also useful to have a pilot program effort before launching a full-scale program. It permits experimentation without too many risks or inconveniences to staff and patients.

Whatever physical space is designated should be carefully delineated as the day hospital area, even if the area only enjoys that distinction two or three days per week. Part of the challenge of creating a therapeutic environment that will maximize the effectiveness of the program for the patients is in giving it a clear-cut identity. That identity begins with the physical facility and the day hospital staff. The integral quality and nature of the program should be evident in every aspect.

The use and design of physical space in program planning and delivery of treatment services will be further determined by the demands and volume of individual treatment services. For example, existing plumbing and wiring may leave no choice as to where physical therapy will be located or where the dining area will be. If an existing physical therapy department is being shared with an inpatient population, its location will be predetermined. The most important guiding principle should be to encourage the independence of patients in moving from one therapy to another. The aim should be for normal patient flow in the designated program area, which, preferably, should be all on one level. Some day hospital patients will be able to wheel themselves or walk aided by assistive devices if their next treatment is within a reasonable distance. Otherwise, assistance by another person will become necessary, and the result will be increasing patient dependence and increased day hospital costs.

Generally, the major areas will consist of public space and administration, medical and nursing, speech therapy, social services, physical therapy, occupational therapy, large group activities and patient dining, staff areas, and miscellaneous services. In arranging functional groupings of these areas, consideration should be given to which services require single-purpose space (such as the physical therapy treatment area), and which, if scheduled properly, can be rendered in a multipurpose space. The same small room would be suitable, for example, for admission interviewing, a social work counseling session, a speech therapy session, or nutrition counseling. A group activities room used from 9 to 11.30 a.m. and 1.30 to 5 p.m. can become a patient dining room between 11.30 a.m. and 1.30 p.m., provided there is housekeeping staff available to clean up and make the necessary changes between sessions.

Cheerful, clean, well-lighted, attractive surroundings are important to the therapeutic environment for patients and staff. A highly motivated and imaginative paid and volunteer staff can create a non-institutional feeling even in the oldest of institutional structures. The physical and mental impairments of patients should be considered in the colors selected, the type of flooring, wall displays, furnishings, the height and contour of chairs, table heights, furniture groupings, and so forth. If necessary, color-coded directional guides can be incorporated in the decorating scheme.

The objectives are to increase the functional independence of the participants, to promote social interaction, to minimize any negative image of an institutional, illness-oriented environment in favor of a positive image, and to reinforce participant expectations for recovery.

### Therapy Space Requirements

Therapy space will be determined by the anticipated daily census and by the specific nature of the treatment program. Staff participation in planning and allocation of space is most useful because they are the most familiar with the utilization patterns, the traffic flow, and with some of the necessary safeguards. A large, attractive activity area will be useless without adequate toilet facilities nearby. Large open areas with many exits would be disastrous for a program that serves a large number of disoriented patients. If there is room for flexibility in space assignments, a major consideration should be the promotion of increasing independence of patients in going from one area to another, making them feel comfortable physically and emotionally and creating a place where they feel they belong. Many of them already feel displaced within their social structure of family and community and are isolated by their limited mobility. A physical structure that minimizes these feelings will provide a therapeutic milieu.

Consideration must also be given to the provision of nonskid flooring, wall railings, good lighting and acoustics, good heat and ventilation. Specific requirements for medical services, and physical and occupational therapy, will be discussed in the appropriate chapters. Social work and speech therapy need both individual rooms and group areas, but they can share the latter.

### Rest Areas

The day hospital has been referred to as a "hospital without beds." The reference is an interesting one, but it is not quite precise. The day hospital is not completely without beds, but it uses the few beds it has somewhat differently from the inpatient hospital. Its beds are most frequently used for brief rest periods for those patients whose physical resources are so limited that they cannot sustain a full day of therapeutic activity.

### Toilet Facilities

A day hospital with a population consisting predominantly of chronically ill, functionally impaired elderly will require toilet areas with all available assistive devices to enable them to be as independent as possible. This will include raised toilet seats, grab bars, and wheelchair accessibility to toilets, basins, and towels or hand dryers. An abundance of toilets will represent an enormous saving in staff time and patient discomfort and indignity.

Bathing and shower facilities will also require special equipment to ensure accessibility. Some day hospitals provide this service as part of personal care services if the patient cannot be showered or bathed at home. Others will only use the facility for demonstrations and for instructing the patient, the family, and/or a home health aide in the procedure.

The breakdown of square footage of floor space in Appendix B demonstrates the requirements for the various areas as outlined in the plans for a day hospital connected with a rehabilitation center. Appendix C shows floor plans for a purpose-built day hospital unit in England.

## CHAPTER THREE

# *Staffing*

The achievement of a day hospital's goals will depend heavily upon the appropriate selection and utilization of its major human resources—namely, its staff. The staff must be committed philosophically and programmatically to the day hospital concept, and their values must be consistent with those of the program administration. An integrated, interdisciplinary approach to patient care must be a concept that is realized, not just theorized. Broadly defined, staffing is a comprehensive personnel function, beginning with the creation of a staff and maintenance of conditions favorable to optimum work performance. In order to deliver quality patient care, decisions must be made concerning the quantity, qualifications, and distribution of staff; adequate provisions must also be made for their orientation, training, and development. Staffing patterns and composition will be influenced by many factors: program objectives and philosophy, the organizational environment in which the program is located, financial and legal constraints, and the availability of other community resources including volunteers. Table 3–1 shows staffing patterns based on average daily attendance.

## ORGANIZATIONAL ENVIRONMENT

The immediate environment in which a day hospital program functions has a significant impact upon its success or failure. The

TABLE 3-1. Staffing Requirements of Adult Day Health Centers
Administered by the State of Washington Department of
Social and Health Services Office on Aging
(January 1978)

*Staffing hours per week according to average daily attendance*

| Staff Position | ADA under 20 | ADA 20–29 | ADA 30–39 | ADA over 40 |
|---|---|---|---|---|
| Director | 30 | 40 | 40 | 40 |
| Registered Nurse | 30 | 40 | 40 | 40 |
| Practical Nurse | — | — | 30 | 40 |
| Social Service Specialist | 30 | 40 | 40 | 40 |
| Assistant Social Service Specialist | — | — | 30 | 40 |
| Activity Coordinator | — | 40 | 40 | 40 |
| Occupational Therapist | 10 | 20 | 40 | 40 |
| Assistant Occupational Therapist | — | — | — | 40 |
| Aide | — | 20 | 40 | 80 |
| Administrative Support | 30 | 40 | 60 | 80 |

establishment of a new patient care unit within an ongoing hospital
program, for example, may add or take away resources from other
units, eliciting support or concern from those tangentially involved.
It may also happen that the existing hospital program may add or
remove resources from a new unit, either helping it to succeed or
making its survival difficult. The environment imposed by the sponsoring organization sets the ground rules for the unit and has a direct
impact upon staff function and their sense of identity. If staff members are primarily identified with services outside the day hospital
unit and no one belongs solely to it, problems are more likely to arise
because of fragmentation of authority and philosophical differences.
Ideally, all units of the sponsoring facility will be working to achieve

patient care goals in the same manner, and there will be no fragmentation. However, the ideal is seldom real, and a conflict of values and goals can become a major obstacle to the administration of a program that is not autonomous and consistent in its method of achieving quality patient care.


## PROGRAM OBJECTIVES

The overall objectives of a day hospital will vary from one community to another and from one provider setting to another, as discussed in Chapter 2. They may be designed to serve a patient population of select age groups, of select diagnostic categories, or of certain degrees of functional impairment. No matter what their particular focus, they are likely to share the following common goals:

1.    to sustain and/or improve the functional capacity of the participants;
2.    to improve the quality of life for the participants;
3.    to provide relief of management for responsible family members;
4.    to avoid inappropriate utilization of other health care resources; and
5.    to increase the availability of community-based options within the health care continuum.

Despite the universality of these objectives, there will be varying degrees of program emphasis, depending upon the treatment needs of the participants, the number of participants, and the actual mix of those being treated. If the number and categories of professional staff are fixed, then it will be necessary to establish limits on the numbers and functional categories of patients who can be treated on a given day. Certain patients, for example, will require individual physical therapy treatments, and some will benefit from group exercise. If the day hospital has only one registered physical therapist, then it will be necessary to determine how many patients of each category can be scheduled in one day. A daily patient sample treatment profile is shown in Table 3-2.

Determining the daily patient capacity of a day hospital is not simply a matter of numbers. It involves making optimal assignments for quality of care. In order to maximize staff resources, it is necessary to consider the tasks being assigned and their complexity before determining staff requirements. "Ambulation training" will be less

**TABLE 3-2. Daily Patient Sample Treatment Profile**

*Daily average based on two days a week*

| Treatment/Service | Patients dependent in 5 to 6 Activities of Daily Living (ADL)[1] | Patients dependent in 2 to 4 Activities of Daily Living (ADL)[1] |
|---|---|---|
| Nursing[2] | 15 minutes | 15 minutes |
| Personal Care[3] | 90 minutes | 45 minutes |
| Social Service[2] | 15 minutes | 30 minutes |
| Physical Therapy | | |
|   Individual | 45 minutes | 45 minutes |
|   Group | 30 minutes | 30 minutes |
| Occupational Therapy | | |
|   Individual | 45 minutes | — |
| Group | — | 45 minutes |
| Speech Therapy[4] | | |
|   Individual | | |
|   Group | | |
| Patient Activities[5] | | |
|   Quiet diversional activities | 45 minutes | 30 minutes |
|   Social interaction and program activities | — | 45 minutes |
| TOTAL TIME | 4 3/4 hours | 4 3/4 hours |

[1] ADL refers to bathing, dressing, toileting, transfer, continence, and feeding
[2] Does not include time spent by nursing and social work staff in coordinating patient care with physicians, family, and outside agencies
[3] Personal care includes assistance at time of arrival and departure and toileting
[4] Not all patients receive speech therapy. Average is 45 minutes
[5] Some patients may be unable to participate in a recreation program. Initially this may be a rest period for some

difficult and less time-consuming for a young disabled fracture patient than for an 85-year-old severe cardiac, ar̸ ̸ritic patient. Individual patient treatment plans and care requ̸ ̸ments must be clearly identified. In addition, supervising personnel must be aware of, and sensitive to, an individual's capacity for accepting workload. The speech therapist who is especially skilled in working with aphasic patients and likes doing this will probably deliver the highest quality of care. In order to determine the specific combination of staff members required, it will be necessary to summarize the treatment needs of the participant population and to relate that summary to the known productivity and commitments of the program staff. There are many ways in which this can be achieved.

A critical analysis of the job functions within each department can be made through a detailed description of tasks. This functional task analysis of each position in combination with a time study will reveal the specific nature of the job and the appropriate amount of time spent in performing the various tasks. An analysis such as that shown in Appendix D will provide the necessary information on staff productivity. A sample analysis of time distribution for the day hospital administrative assistant in transportation appears in Appendix E.

The functional task analysis and time study must then be matched with the treatment needs analyses of the patient population in order to quantify staffing requirements, establish the patient-staff ratio, and design treatment schedules. This analysis can also be useful in redefining or realigning staff roles, setting unit costs, and budgeting for specific service cost centers. It can also serve as documentation for requested changes in reimbursement rates or in rate setting. It should provide the baseline data for many mangement decisions, lead to better communication among team members providing care, and to more effective staff assignments. Staff requirements for adult day care centers in California are shown in Appendix F.

Whether for purposes of time study, staff ratio analysis, or routine management planning, there must be a clear-cut definition of job roles, with room for some flexibility built into that definition. Defining staff roles and planning how time is going to be utilized will always include planning for potential "dead time." Supplemental tasks that can fill such time spaces should be delegated in advance. Another solution is utilizing a talented staff member in a dual capacity when time permits. This requires managerial recognition and encouragement of staff potential. It not only provides job enrichment for the individual, but also permits career exploration.

erefore, it is important that a staff member have a personality that
ily and constructively engages with the elderly. Flexibility in
proach to the elderly is beneficial, and those who offer only a rigid
ponse to the older person should be excluded. In order to care for
e aging, in whom insecurity is prevalent, personnel must be secure
emselves.

A requirement for working with a day hospital patient should
e a strong conviction that he is rehabilitative. In this effort, all of
ie elderly person's constructive possibilities are to be supported and
nhanced, not just his physical being. A staff member's constant
ncouragement and patience are significant in enabling the patient to
chieve optimum physical and psychosocial functioning. Many long-
erm care personnel who have been trained in an institutional setting
iave a stronger orientation to the illness of patients than to their
wellness. The day hospital emphasizes the positive aspects of the
patients' health and aims to increase their independence.

## HUMAN RESOURCES

To remain healthy and efficient, an organization must continually evaluate how it is using its staff members' potentials. Members
of a therapeutic environment who are not permitted to exercise
the full range of their abilities, or whose competence is not recognized,
are likely to become discouraged and disinterested. An important
part of the environment is a program that permits all members to
grow by encouraging them to develop skills and techniques and by
helping them to increase their knowledge. Each staff member should
be not only encouraged, but expected to fulfill his potential as a
therapeutic agent. Training resources are important for staff orientation, staff development, and staff retention. All training should be
focused upon updating knowledge, upgrading skills, and tapping the
existing wealth of knowledge and experience within all staff. The
overall goals, of course, are to improve quality of care and increase
the job satisfaction of those who are delivering the care. Formal
cross-disciplinary staff orientation, in-service education, increased
accessibility to other agency educational programs, tuition refund
plans, encouraged participation at professional conferences, opportunities to supervise students, and encouragement of upward
career mobility and individually initiated program ideas are but a few
of the necessary approaches to training. Financial provision for such
programs should be included in budget planning.

## MULTIDISCIPLINARY TEAM CONCEPT

Rehabilitation is a unique program in medical
it requires such a wide spectrum of skills. The rehabili
in a day hospital is truly an interdisciplinary effort
achieved by a multidisciplinary team of health profe
social workers, physical therapists, occupational thera
and speech therapists—and paraprofessionals, und
supervision of a physician. They are all necessary t
integration of the patient into the community. The
ment programs of each discipline are discussed else
book, but the day-to-day functioning of the multidis
is a staffing concern.

The team leader may be the physician, a nurse, a
or one of the other professionals. The physician may be
a part-time basis and not willing nor able to assume the
ship responsibility. Any individual professional who pos
interpersonal skills, administrative abilities, and a genu
ment to the program's philosophy and objectives w
make a competent team leader. In addition to having a
standing of the interdisciplinary nature of the rehabilitati
the team leader must provide the kind of leadership that w
and structure the unit as a therapeutic reality. It is essen
effective operation of a team leader that those members o
whose activities he or she coordinates and who are not dire
his or her supervision recognize his or her authority to cc
The leadership role will be assumed by different individuals at
times, depending upon the immediate goal of a particular sta
Titles will vary, but for organizational purposes, the le
responsibility should be clearly delineated.

The patients' needs are so varied and comprehensive that e
treatment requires a true blending of staff skills, with eac
member relinquishing a certain amount of autonomy for the
good of the patients. This requires staff who are personal
professionally secure and genuinely concerned with delivering
ity patient care; these personality traits are as crucial to q
care as are professional skills and competence. It is essential
the team members share a compatible set of values, experie
and goals; it is the team leader's responsibility to inspire a
tinuing focus upon these goals.

Although a day hospital treating adults will encompass all a
it will undoubtedly have a larger proportion of elderly participa

Staff training should be made available to paraprofessional, clerical, and administrative support staff as well as to professional staff. Specific skills training on the job or at another location should be aimed at increasing employee competence and expanding their vocational and avocational horizons. On-the-job training programs for paraprofessionals funded through the Department of Labor have enabled day hospitals to train nursing assistants as occupational therapy aides, electrocardiograph technicians, laboratory assistants, and geriatric technicians. Within the same funding mechanism, entry level clerks have become medical secretaries, medical record assistants, and medical assistants, following formal training in medical terminology and office practice combined with on-the-job training.

Skilled professionals with many years of clinical experience may not have had the advantage of management training, nor on-the-job experience in that area. Some will benefit from supervision and training in how to teach, whether it is in patient education, consumer education, or in teaching paraprofessionals. These new skills will make them more valuable as staff members and will permit more varied assignments within their jobs.

Staff participation in program planning should be encouraged. Their ideas for improving patient care are founded upon practical experience and should be given serious consideration. Formal communication channels should be established through staff conferences and team meetings. Opportunities should also be provided to teach team members how to communicate with each other. Staff also need to be trained to participate in decision making and in decision implementation.

## FINANCIAL AND LEGAL CONSTRAINTS

Financial constraints that affect central staffing will include budgetary limits as well as reimbursement mechanisms. Reimbursement formulas very often dictate the staffing levels. For example, Medicare reimbursement will be approved for physical therapy if the treatment is given or supervised directly by a registered physical therapist. Local, state, and federal policies relevant to reimbursement will require careful analysis in program planning and staffing.

In certain states, adult day health services are regulated by a single state agency, and monitoring includes physical space requirements, patient eligibility, treatment program, staffing, and fees.

Samples for the staffing regulations for two states appear in Table 3-1 and Appendix F.

## COMMUNITY RESOURCES, INCLUDING VOLUNTEERS

Some of the needed services may be provided to participants by other community agencies through a contractual arrangement. Some day care programs have obtained services of public health nurses, dentists, consulting physicians, medical specialists, audiologists, and so forth, in this manner, since the demand for these services may not be consistent. The decision to utilize such resources may be based on the limited demand, or the availablity of better service, or the cost-effectiveness of the arrangement. Some of the disadvantages of such an arrangement are the time and effort required in coordinating staff services from several sources within different administrative structures, the potential danger of reduced quality assurance, and the possibility of a more loosely knit team approach. However, all of these factors must be weighed within the organizational priorities of the program and the budgetary constraints.

Volunteers are one of the greatest community resources, and they can play an important role in the staffing of a day hospital, provided certain safeguards are taken. The commitment that volunteers bring to the program and their interest in the well-being of the patients are factors that accord the program added status and can enhance the self-image of patients. In any long-term setting, one of the goals is to reduce the isolation of the patients and to help them relate better to the community. The social interaction with volunteers is one way in which this can be achieved, and the very presence of volunteers tells the patients that the community is interested in them. However, as with all staff—paid or volunteer—their recruitment, selection, orientation, appropriate assignment, training, supervision, and recognition are crucial to success.

Volunteers may be recruited through local volunteer service bureaus, churches, schools, colleges, service clubs, senior citizen organizations, professional organizations, newspaper articles, and through personal contacts made by staff members and by patients' families. An interview with the staff member responsible for volunteers should cover in great detail the volunteer's personal goals in volunteering, opportunities available, qualifications needed, supervision provided, as well as specific hours and schedule. Very often, an individual applicant will have special skills and interests that are not currently available in the program but could be added. It is important to offer the potential volunteers ample opportunity to share their aims and expectations and to establish channels for ongoing communication and mutual evaluation.

Part of the selection process should include, if possible, ample opportunity for observation by the applicant. A trial experience as a program assistant will permit the volunteer to get a job sample without any obligation. Although well motivated, some volunteers find that working with severely impaired individuals is too depressing. Others may be inclined to increase a patient's dependency because they are too eager to help or too impatient to wait and let the individual help himself. Unless they have had prior experience in working with a group of such patients, there would be no way for them to know their response to these situations. A trial experience is usually appreciated.

It is equally true that some individuals will be fearful or timid about working with the chronically ill or disabled. An orientation period that can include some information about the nature of chronic illnesses, the resulting disabilities, specific illustrations of how volunteers can help, the type of on-the-job training and supervision that will be available, and so forth, will increase their feelings of adequacy. Usually, experienced volunteers who can serve as role models will be the most convincing and persuasive speakers.

It is common to have mature women seeking volunteer jobs as a means of gaining "recent experience" or sampling a "second career" before seeking paid employment. This motivation should be explored openly, and the applicant should be assisted in determining whether this is a realistic goal.

> Mrs. G., a professional social worker, came to the day hospital seeking volunteer work in the Social Work Department. When asked why she was not seeking paid employment as an M.S.S.W., she replied that she had not worked in a number of years, the job market was very tight, and she wanted only part-time work. The interviewer then asked whether she was hoping eventually to find permanent paid employment in the day hospital, and Mrs. G. said that that was certainly her top goal. When she learned that no part-time social work would ever be possible, she became uninterested in volunteering.

Volunteer employment represents a substantial investment for all concerned, and this investment should be discussed and considered in the selection of volunteers. The individual who is self-sufficient and possesses skills that can be easily introduced into the program (such as a typist, a receptionist, a friendly visitor, a guitarist) will be useful even on a short-term basis. But one could not justify selection on a short-term basis of a person who is going to require a great deal of guidance, close supervision, and considerable on-the-job training by a paid staff member.

### Volunteer Assignments

The tasks assigned to volunteers will be governed by the day hospital program aims and needs, the volunteer's skills and needs, and the aims and supervisory skills of a specific department head. Many health professionals have not had the benefit of a positive experience with volunteer staff, and some find it difficult to supervise volunteer or even paid staff members.

The coordinator of volunteers will need time and skill in determining appropriate assignments. It is important for everyone concerned—particularly the patient—that this be a successful experience.

Volunteer groups such as scouting or service organizations will sometimes accept a group assignment. For example, a local woman's club has operated and staffed a day hospital patient notion shop two mornings a week; a chairperson shopped for the items and scheduled her club volunteers to work one or two mornings a month. She also arranged for sending substitutes when someone was absent. A Senior Scout group has provided day hospital tray favors two or three days prior to any major holiday. A Junior Red Cross group has arranged the entertainment for monthly patient birthday parties.

The number and variety of assignments are limitless, depending upon the skills and motivation of the staff, the coordinator, and the volunteers.

### Training and Supervision of Volunteers

Volunteers, like paid staff, want to improve their skills, update their knowledge, and generally increase their adequacy in job performance. The coordinator of volunteers can work with the assigned supervisor of a particular volunteer to determine how this can best be achieved. A lending library of pertinent journal articles and pamphlets would be one source, while program announcements and invitations to relevant lectures, in-service education, and so on, would be another. Encouraging volunteers to participate in case conferences, when appropriate, provides an opportunity for them to share their observations of a patient and in addition get feedback on patient progress from others. Qualified volunteers are also excellent training resource personnel.

Mrs. B. is an experienced volunteer speech therapy aide who has enjoyed success in conducting current events groups with speech impaired patients in the day hospital. Since many volunteers have had little or no experience in dealing with this type of patient, Mrs. B. offered to teach them ways of communicating effectively.

Professional supervision and training are essential if one is going to use volunteers in a day hospital. It protects the patient, the day hospital, the supervisor, and the volunteer. It enables volunteers to improve and to evaluate their own job performance and is likely to increase their job satisfaction.

### Recognition of Volunteers

Volunteer recognition does not begin nor end with a ceremony, certificates, or tea parties. Annual recognition of this kind is important in that it permits other hospital staff, trustees, and the community to learn about and pay tribute to the contribution made by the volunteer staff. But "recognition" must happen daily, in the way volunteers are received, accepted, and made aware of appreciation for their valuable contribution. It is simply a matter of according them the same dignity and courtesy that everyone would like to receive in all human relations.

MAUREEN A. RYAN

## CHAPTER FOUR

# Patient Admissions and Discharges

## ELIGIBILITY CRITERIA

In order to function as a new health care option and to achieve its goal of rehabilitation, it is essential that the day hospital admit only those patients who are appropriate, and that it refer to more suitable community resources those patients who do not meet the admission criteria. To accomplish this goal, criteria to determine eligibility must be established, as well as a process that makes the services being offered accessible to those requiring them. Eligibility criteria will vary from one setting to another, but basically they should serve to define and delimit the scope of services of the program.

For such a definition to be achieved, all disciplines and departments must participate in establishing the criteria. One of the roles of administration will be to establish the amount and kind of resources it can make available to each discipline. It can, for example, allocate the amount of space and money that is available for equipment for the physical therapy department, but the physical therapist in charge must then define the treatment modalities that can be provided within those limitations. If there is inadequate space and plumbing for hydrotherapy, patients requiring that treatment modality must be eliminated from the program, or arrangements must be made for them to receive those treatments elsewhere. Once each discipline has established the scope of service it can provide, all members of the interdisciplinary treatment team must have an opportunity to contribute to the development of each of the admission criteria. There must be a general consensus on the philosophy, objectives, and extent of services of the program if there is to be a coordinated and comprehensive approach to the rehabilitation of participants.

The following are criteria of one day hospital program:

1. *Age:* Adult, 14 years old or older.
2. *Financial:* Capable of paying for the services rendered by the day hospital.
3. *Transportation:* Capable of being transported to the day hospital. Can provide own transportation, or is eligible for the service as provided by the day hospital.
4. *Medical:* The individual must be under the care of a physician, or under the medical surveillance of a clinic or neighborhood health center. The physician must approve the individual's application to the day hospital and provide the day hospital with information related to the patient's medical condition prior to admission. The physician must be willing to continue to be the primary provider of medical care while the applicant participates in the day hospital program.
5. *Functional:* The applicant's performance in mobility, activities of daily living, and communication can be improved through a therapeutic program including physical, occupational, and speech therapy, medical surveillance, nursing services, and psychosocial support and counseling. Generally the applicant will be characterized by the following:
   a. Nonambulatory, with the potential, after a course of individualized therapy including ambulation training, for one of the following:
      (1) independent ambulation;
      (2) independent ambulation with assistive device;
      (3) ambulation with assistive device and observation by another;
      (4) independent in a wheelchair.
   b. Dependent in one or more of the following activities of daily living:
      (1) grooming;
      (2) bathing;
      (3) toileting;
      (4) feeding;
      (5) homemaking (including meal planning and preparation, work simplification, and housekeeping chores);
      (6) taking medications;

(7)  making contact via telephone to meet needs;

(8)  dressing.

After a course of individualized treatment and training in activities of daily living, has the potential for:

(1)  independence in the deficient areas;

(2)  independence with assistive devices and observation and/or cueing by another;

(3)  independence with assistive devices, or performance of these activities with the assistance of another who has been trained in these skills.

 c. Handicapped in his ability to comprehend verbal and written instructions and/or in his ability to express himself.

6.  *Behavioral:*

 a. Cannot require more supervision than the day hospital can provide to ensure his safety while attending the program.

 b. Must be capable of participation in the treatment program.

 c. Must be willing to participate in the treatment program.

7.  *Social:* The applicant's behavior or manners must be acceptable in a group setting or amenable to modification.

8.  *Environment:* The applicant must have adequate resources within his home environment to assure his safety and to ensure that the objectives of the day hospital can be met.

References have been made in the criteria to the candidate's ability and willingness to participate in the program. This may be interpreted as an attempt to assess the candidate's motivation. However, it would be better to assume that all applicants either are or can be motivated. It is assumed that they want to be well or more functional than they are, and that the day hospital must help those who apply and are eligible to achieve that goal.

### ADMISSION PROCESS

The admission process should be designed with as few encumbrances as possible. Those seeking admission should not feel that their first major task is to figure out how to break through the red tape, but rather how to use their energy for their major objective, namely, "to get well." The admission process is depicted in the flow chart in Appendix G.

The admissions director is in a key position and must be chosen with extreme care. He or she should be mature, responsible, intelligent, thoughtful, tactful, attentive to details, considerate of others, present a good appearance, and be skilled in effective communication. Although these are the qualities desirable in *every* staff member, they are particularly important for an admissions director. This person is usually the patient's and his family's initial contact with the day hospital and is important in setting the tone for the duration of the patient's stay. He must work closely with many people of diverse ages, cultural backgrounds, educational preparations, life experiences, and orientation.

Several factors must be considered when space is allocated for the admissions office. It should be located near the building entrance and as close as possible to the transportation office. In addition to a working office, the director of admissions should have a room available for patient and family interviews; this should be sufficiently large to accommodate a patient in a wheelchair, several staff members, and several family members.

The admission process begins with the initial inquiry. The majority of inquiries are made by telephone and come from professionals in the health care community, such as physicians, nurses, and social workers. Many also come from the community at large. It is imperative that all inquiries be channeled to one individual, the admissions director, who is well informed about the eligibility criteria, the services provided, and charges. By posing certain questions to the inquirer, the potential of the candidate can generally be ascertained, and, when appropriate, an application is sent. Usually additional applications will be sent to health care professionals to facilitate further referrals.

The application has two parts. One is sent to the individual to obtain sociodemographic and financial data; the other is sent to the individual's physician requesting medical data. If the request for admission comes from someone other than the physician, a covering letter and information explaining the program is sent along with the request for medical information. The form requests historical and current medical information and indication from the physician concerning the services required by the patient. This, in effect, becomes the physician's order for assessment of need for service. Once the patient has been assessed and deemed eligible, the day hospital physician will write the orders for the rehabilitation treatment regimen. No one is admitted without the consent and recommendations of his personal physician. The goal should be to reinforce and augment the role of the primary physician via the services provided. Examples of application forms are shown in Appendix H.

When the applications are returned to the admissions office, the candidate is given an appointment for a preadmission interview. Generally, the candidate comes to the day hospital for the interview, but he may be seen in the acute hospital or at his home if necessary. At the time of the interview, the admissions director establishes financial eligibility. Approximate fees will be determined by the amount and kind of services the individual may need. This will be established once the nurse has conducted the interview. Reimbursement policies of third-party payers are explained as well as the approximate share for which the participant himself will be responsible. The ability of the candidate and/or his family to provide transportation is explored, and various options, including the transportation service of the day hospital, are explained. The admissions director also explains the nature of the program and the scope of services.

The nurse who will be the case manager, should the applicant be admitted, conducts an interview to determine whether or not the admission criteria pertain. That is, she will make a professional judgment as to whether or not the applicant's functional status can be improved or whether his care at home can be improved. She will also determine whether day hospital treatment is appropriate and that services required are not presently being provided by other agencies or individuals. The day hospital physician may be consulted when admissibility is uncertain. Suggested guidelines for the preadmission interview are given in Appendix J.

If the applicant is admissible, the physical and psychosocial problems that seem amenable to intervention are discussed with the applicant and his family. A tentative treatment plan is outlined, date of admission and frequency of attendance are determined, costs of service are reviewed, and, if necessary, transportation is arranged. If the applicant is not admissible, an attempt is made to direct the individual to more appropriate sources of care. The referral source is advised of findings, actions taken, and alternative care recommendations. The applicant's personal physician is sent a written report.

Between the patient's acceptance and actual admission, many details must be managed. Sometimes additional information about the patient's health status comes to light in the preadmission interview, requiring the acquisition of additional records. Often several phone calls must be made and numerous forms completed to satisfy the reimbursement procedure. Additional questions, generated by the preadmission interview, may mean phone calls from the patient or his family.

Ideally, all disciplines participate in the development of the philosophy, objectives, and eligibility criteria of the day hospital program. This may not be feasible at the outset. It may take some time for the staff to work together and develop the mutual respect for each other's contribution to the rehabilitation effort before this occurs. When this is accomplished, staff may also be ready to permit one individual to screen candidates for admission. All candidates are admitted conditionally. That is, each discipline, including the physician, reserves its decision on whether a candidate is appropriate until a comprehensive assessment is completed. It is after this assessment that the orders for treatment are written and treatment begun. Few candidates have been found unacceptable after they have passed the rigors of the preadmission screening. On the day of admission, the first evaluation should be that of the physician. The assessment process is discussed in detail in another chapter and outlined in Appendix I.

### DATA COLLECTION

A great deal of information is channeled through an admissions office. Much of the information must be retained in a particular format to satisfy state and federal regulatory agencies and third-party payers. Uniform data, recorded daily and compiled into monthly, quarterly, and annual reports, can be used for many different purposes. The information collected will serve as a basis for an overall evaluation of the program's effectiveness and for initiating any changes that may be required to meet the needs of applicants and of the community being served.

Admission data collection should include the number and source of community inquiries and the results of those inquiries. An analysis of those patients judged inadmissible and the reasons for their ineligibility will indicate areas of community need not being served by the day hospital. Review of the geographic location of inquiries and admissions will give some indication of the success of community outreach and the result of patient recruitment efforts. Reports should also include current census average daily attendance, admissions and discharges, pay class of patients, and primary diagnoses. (See Appendix H for samples of various application, admission, medical information, and census forms).

The most important measure of a rehabilitation program's effectiveness is the functional improvement of its patients. The functional status of the patient is recorded upon admission in a uniform, systematic fashion, and again at the time of periodic reevaluations. The same criteria must be applied prior to discharge in order to measure the degree of improvement. The refinement of these measures and the use of uniform definitions of functional status will permit useful analyses and program comparisons. (A sample of such a reporting system used by the State of California appears in Appendix R.)

## DISCHARGE PLANNING

The same objectives should be considered when planning the discharge process. In fact, the process should begin with the preadmission interview. The candidate and his family should understand on what basis he is being admitted, what goals are to be accomplished, and on what basis he may continue to participate in the program. The patient and his family should also be involved in the plans for discharge. Discharge criteria must be acceptable to the physician, staff, patient, and family. Plans for discharge must be coordinated. This may be the function of the nurse (case manager), the social worker, or any combination of the rehabilitation staff necessary to effect an easy transition for the patient. It is important that the patient's primary physician receive reports of the patient's progress and be involved in the discharge plans. In addition to reports of the patient's progress in the program, the primary physician should receive a report on patient status at the time of discharge.

### Discharge Criteria

The following is an example of one day hospital's discharge criteria. A participant at the day hospital will be discharged when:

1. The goals of the treatment plan as established by the team and patient have been achieved, are realized to be unattainable, or if realistic goals cannot be established by the team.
2. The participant's physician withdraws him from the program.
3. The participant's condition warrants more treatment than can be provided by the day hospital.
4. The participant's condition does not require the comprehensive services provided by the day hospital.
5. The participant is unable or unwilling to participate in the treatment program.
6. The environment in which the participant resides is hazardous to his safety.
7. Transportation can no longer be provided.
8. Payment for services is not made within a reasonable period.

ROBERT C. OLIVER

## CHAPTER FIVE

# *Patient Transportation*

A safe, dependable, efficient, and comfortable system of transportation is indispensable to the day hospital's effective operation. Among the alternative methods of transport that may be utilized to achieve this goal are: transportation provided by the day hospital or its sponsoring facility; a public specialized transportation service; a nonprofit, community-sponsored specialized transportation service; commercial vendors whose main business is the transportation of disabled persons; private taxi companies for patients who are not wheelchair-bound; transportation by volunteers, family members, or friends of patients. Usually a combination of several methods will be necessary.

### VEHICLE STANDARDS

Regardless of which method(s) of transportation is decided upon, the day hospital should require assurance from the provider that the following considerations are being met:

1. fulfillment of requirements for state inspection and any other necessary governmental regulations;
2. adequate liability insurance coverage;
3. regular maintenance checks on all equipment and vehicles;

4.  provision of safety equipment such as safe, convenient loading and unloading steps, ramps, or hydraulic lifts and floor locks for wheelchairs to ensure stability and security during locomotion;
5.  adequate heating and cooling systems for extreme weather conditions;
6.  two-way radio communication equipment;
7.  flexibility of interior vehicle arrangement to allow for a changing variety of disability requirements;
8.  good visibility to permit passengers maximum enjoyment of the outside world;
9.  careful selection and training of drivers.

Guidelines for modes of transportation that can be used by patients with various medical conditions are shown in Appendix K.

### GEOGRAPHIC CONSIDERATIONS

The catchment area of a day hospital is governed by the travel time required from the patient's residence to the facility. Travel time one way from the outer limits should average about one hour and should never exceed one and one half hours. The time factor involved in providing the needed physical assistance to move the patient from his home to the vehicle should be included in any time estimates. The fragile physical and emotional condition of the patients attending a day hospital precludes excessive periods spent in transport service vehicles. Although occasional delays will occur because of inclement weather, special traffic conditions, or vehicle breakdown, frequent disruption of patient arrival schedules cannot be tolerated.

### SCHEDULING

The entire professional team in the day hospital is ready and waiting each day for the arrival of the patients. The arrival, as well as the departure, of the patients should be carefully scheduled in accordance with the treatment plans worked out for each individual. Therefore, it is essential that patients be brought by the transportation service on a definite timetable worked out between the transportation administrative assistant at the day hospital and the dispatchers of the transportation vendor. The schedule must be adhered to as rigidly as possible. Delays in arrival disrupt the treatment schedules and become expensive in terms of unused professional staff time and loss of income for patient treatments. Patients become frustrated and anxious when treatments are missed. In some cases, it may result in their missing breakfast, a source of nutrition and socialization. Furthermore, interrupted schedules work considerable hardship on disabled patients who may have to arise two or three hours before the van comes for them in order to be dressed and ready. They are left wondering what has happened and whether or not they are going to get to the day hospital at all that day. For many patients, participation in the day hospital program is their only relief from enforced isolation. Delayed schedules are also very inconvenient for family members or friends who provide the home care for patients. It may mean that they will not be able to go to work that day, or they may not get that period of needed relief from caring for the severely disabled relative or friend.

The larger the catchment area and/or the number of patients, the more complex is the scheduling. Depending on the capability of the transportation vendors serving the day hospital, it may be necessary to schedule patients from certain sections of the catchment area two days a week and from other sections on alternate days of the week. The challenge is in matching distances to be traveled, number of patients to be transported, individual patient therapy schedules, area traffic patterns, road conditions, alternative emergency routes, etc. If a number of vendors are providing the service, there is the added problem of coordinating them and their individual constraints that may be imposed by other commitments, such as school busing handicapped children at specific hours. (An illustration of the catchment area for one day hospital in New York State appears in Appendix L.)

### STAFFING

If the day hospital provides its own transportation, staffing will include the transportation manager, drivers, and vehicle maintenance crew. In some cases drivers may also maintain the vehicles. The manager will supervise the drivers, schedule patient transportation, and act as dispatcher. The manager should be someone experienced in transportation and knowledgeable about the catchment area, since the job responsibilities involved do not permit on-the-job training for a beginner. When transportation is being provided by a number of different vendors, including individual arrangements made by families of patients, an administrative assistant is needed to coordinate patient transportation. This individual might report to either the clinical coordinator or the admissions director, since they must work closely together in order to achieve a smooth operation. (A sample of the time study and tasks of an administrative assistant in transportation appears in Appendix E.)

### PHYSICAL SPACE AND EQUIPMENT

If transportation is provided directly by the day hospital, special vehicles and a garage will be needed. Back-up vehicles for emergency situations and any necessary repair equipment must also be available.

A small office is needed for the manager or administrative assistant, preferably adjacent to or adjoining the admissions office. An area close to the entrance should be designated for patients arriving and awaiting departure, with a small reception area where the administrative assistant can monitor arrivals and departures and where outer clothing can be hung. Wheelchair storage in this area, with adequate security, is most convenient since patients normally transfer to wheelchairs provided by the transportation vendor just prior to departure. A conveniently located lavatory will permit the transportation assistant to assist patients who require help without leaving the general area.

### TRANSPORTATION COSTS AND REIMBURSEMENT

Transportation is likely to be one of the more expensive items in the package of day hospital services. Vendors require a certain return per vehicle in order to meet their profit goals, so it is wise to determine what that return is when contracting for service. By working cooperatively with the vendor in the scheduling process, the day hospital administrator can influence the number of patients who can be transported per day in a single vehicle. Knowing this price will also be useful in reviewing transportation bids. However, if there are not many vendors who transport physically disabled individuals, then containment of transportation costs will be difficult because of the limited competition for the contract. In those states where regulatory agencies do not limit the profit margin of such transportation vendors, prices will tend to be unreasonable.

In negotiating bids on transportation contracts, a careful investigation of potential vendors must be made, directed at areas such as whether or not there are adequately trained drivers and the vendor's record of punctuality, safety performance, and reliability in transporting large groups of patients on a daily basis. Financial stability is also of special importance. This can be checked through the vendors's audited annual statements. New companies sometimes purchase a fleet of vehicles using the contract in lieu of collateral; or they may use the contract to gain licensing from a regulatory agency. It is not advisable to contract under such risks if that contract represents the means of transportation for the majority of the day hospital patients. Major sources of information in such an investigation are discussions with the vendors themselves, in-depth interviews with other health care facilities who have used the potential vendors for a substantive period of time, and licensing agencies.

Reimbursement for transportation must be explored with individuals' insurance carriers at the time of admission. Medicare does not recognize transportation for outpatient-type services at the present time, but it is reimbursable for Medicaid-eligible patients. In some communities, local service clubs or community agencies will finance the transportation of individual patients. In other cases, they have purchased vehicles for use by a day hospital. The transportation office encourages families to pool together in the use of a private taxi for patients from the same geographic area, thus making it less costly. The need for more universal recognition of transportation as a service essential to the delivery of day hospital care is an area for continuing effort on the part of day hospital advocates.

MAUREEN A. RYAN

## CHAPTER SIX

# Patient Assessment and Treatment Planning

If the focus of a day hospital program is to assist an individual to achieve his highest level of functioning, emphasizing independence in activities of daily living, then the objectives of the program are:

1. to promote restoration of function and prevent progressive disability and deterioration;
2. to assist in the psychosocial adjustment to chronic illness and/or disability;
3. to assist the participant in utilizing his strength to maintain a level of wellness within the limitations imposed by his illness and/or disability;
4. to redirect energies in a manner consistent with limitations to satisfy social and recreational needs.

In order to plan and implement a program that will achieve these objectives, each client should participate in a comprehensive interdisciplinary health assessment. The purpose of this comprehensive assessment is to identify those problems that interfere with the individual's ability to reach his maximum adaptive state. Those participating in the assessment process should include:

1. the client;
2. the client's family or "significant others";

3. the client's primary physician;
4. the day hospital physician;
5. nursing staff;
6. registered physical therapist;
7. registered occupational therapist;
8. speech pathologist;
9. social worker;
10. nutritional consultant.

The assessment process actually begins prior to admission, when the physical and psychosocial health status of the applicant is reviewed by the nurse and a temporary problem list is constructed with suggested interventions. Upon admission, the client's status is evaluated by each discipline focusing on its particular area of expertise. The multidisciplinary evaluation consists of:

1. *Psychosocial assessment* by a social worker, based on an interview with the client and a member of the family to determine whether emotional, social, spiritual, environmental, or financial stress may be interfering with the individual's adaptive abilities.
2. *Nursing assessment* to evaluate current health status (includes completion of the health history and physical examination) and the individual's ability to cope with his illness physically and psychologically.
3. *Medical evaluation.* Generally, the nursing assessment that includes a physical examination is the first evaluation performed on admission. At the time of evaluation, the day hospital physician reviews the history and physical findings and contributes to the overall health plan by designating which protocols are to be followed in the medical surveillance of the patient.
4. *Physical therapy assessment* to evaluate joint range of motion, muscle strength, gait pattern, and need for prosthetic or orthotic evaluation.
5. *Occupational therapy assessment* to determine the individual's ability to perform activities of daily living, his dexterity, grasp strength, and whether or not sensation, position in space, stereognosis, and perception are intact.
6. *Speech and hearing assessment* to determine the individual's communication skills and to identify speech/language/voice disorders such as aphasia, apraxia, or dysarthria. An audiometric screening is performed to identify hearing impairments.
7. *Nutritional assessment* to determine the adequacy of the

individual's diet and to identify needs related to nutritional counseling, diet planning, and diet supervision.

These assessments may be completed on the day of admission, but it is more likely that they will require two days. The client's endurance and stamina must be considered; if the patient is unduly fatigued, the evaluations will not be truly reflective of his strengths and weaknesses. Upon completion of its evaluation, each discipline outlines the problems identified, goals, a plan for intervention (including specific treatment modalities) that will facilitate achievement of the goals, and an approximate timetable for the achievement of these goals. The client is examined, and the evaluations are reviewed by the day hospital physician, who then authorizes the treatment plan. The staff who constitute the treatment team meet to discuss and share their findings. It is important that each discipline reinforce the efforts of every other discipline if the rehabilitation process is to achieve lasting results.

## THERAPEUTIC MILIEU

Patients usually participate in the day hospital program for from five to six hours during the course of a day. They may spend only four hours in actual treatment, and the rest of the time may be accounted for in going to treatment areas, resting or recreation, mealtime activities, and toileting. This time and these activities can also be considered therapeutic if all staff, including aides and secretaries, are aware of the goals for each patient. This means that everyone must know what the patient is capable of doing for himself, what he is learning to do for himself, and what needs to be done for him. The rehabilitation effort is more effective if the individual greeting the patient on arrival in the morning knows that he is in a wheelchair because it is safer for him to be transported in that manner but that, in fact, he can walk for short distances by himself. At that point, the wheelchair should be taken from him. If the patient is able to remove his own jacket or coat, he should be expected to do so. It would be a disservice to assist him. However, the patient who cannot perform this activity should be assisted immediately and not frustrated or jeopardized by something he is not able to do.

In the same way, a patient who needs to practice a particular gait pattern and to increase his endurance should be encouraged to walk from one activity to another. His schedule must permit the time to do this. He should not be taken in a wheelchair from one therapy to another simply because it is faster and easier for staff to do it for him. The same is true for the patient participating in a speech program. The patient should be encouraged to express himself as often as possible in the manner in which he is most capable. If the patient can only respond with "yes" and "no," then the conversation should be conducted on that level. He should not be asked open-ended questions to which he cannot respond. If the patient is practicing sentences, he should be encouraged in the physical or occupational therapy departments, or even at lunch, to speak in sentences.

It is essential that staff members consider and utilize the overall treatment plan in their interactions with patients. In doing this, patients will achieve a higher and more meaningful level of function in a shorter period of time. The ultimate goal is for patients to function as independently as possible in their own homes. They will first learn and then practice skills in the therapeutic environment. The critical test is whether these skills can be applied in the home setting. The treatment plan is a vital tool in helping patients to achieve this level of independent and purposeful function.

Creating and sustaining an environment that contributes therapeutically to the patient's treatment objectives demands careful consideration. For example, it is important that when the patient enters the treatment area, he feels that he has been expected, that all is in readiness for his arrival, and that his needs have been anticipated. The chronically ill, disabled adult has many concerns and anxieties that can be relieved by knowing that the people who are assisting understand his needs.

## RECORDING

Treatments must be recorded when they are rendered. Progress may not be in evidence after each session, but it should be noted when it occurs. A monthly update should include the patient's level of function, progress toward goals, and the plan for continued treatment. Any change in the patient's status should be recorded as it occurs, and any alterations in the treatment plan brought about as a result of change in the patient should be noted carefully in the patient's medical record.

## TEAM CONFERENCES

Informal communications among the treatment team must occur on a frequent basis, perhaps even daily in some situations. However, it is important to establish some schedule for formal communication about patients' status.

A formal conference schedule that requires each discipline to report on the patient's progress and to record its updated plan of care will facilitate utilization review. The day hospital physician should participate in the conferences, as it is an ideal way for him to review patient progress. Following the conference, the patient should be scheduled for reexamination by the physician to validate the need for continued service.

## REASSESSMENT

Throughout the patient's participation in the program, his status will be continually reassessed to ensure that progress is being made toward reasonable and practical goals.

When patients present problems that cannot be discussed adequately in the forum of the ongoing team conferences, in-depth case conferences should be set up. In these meetings, all pertinent data is reviewed with particular attention to revising the plan; goals are reformulated and new approaches to treatment outlined.

Patients whose treatment may continue beyond three months should be reassessed at three-month intervals. The reassessment should focus on specific measures of function and be compared to the initial evaluation. It is helpful if each discipline develops a system for recording those measures. For example, if a patient is receiving treatment to increase his grasp strength, his actual grasp strength in pounds should be recorded on initial evaluation and again when he is reassessed.

Patients who have been discharged from the program, but whose functional level is expected to change, should be accorded the opportunity to return periodically for a reassessment. This may demonstrate a need for additional service.

Throughout the patient's participation in the program he should be included in the planning and in the setting of goals, and he should be aware of the criteria that mark his progress. The patient's personal physician should receive reports of the initial findings and treatment plan as well as progress reports, and every effort should be made to encourage his participation in the rehabilitation effort.

MAUREEN A. RYAN

## CHAPTER SEVEN

# Medical and Nursing Services

While medicine and nursing are two very separate and distinct disciplines, there is close collaboration between the two within the day hospital in order to achieve the goals of rehabilitation. Their primary responsibility is the health status of the participants. The physical abilities and functional limitations of each participant must be determined before any treatment is initiated, and their status must be monitored closely throughout their participation in the program. It should be remembered that while the thrust of rehabilitation treatment may be to retrain and reeducate the patient's muscles to function more effectively, most patients are still recovering from one or more acute insults to various organs of their bodies, and their medical condition is unstable. Even though a great deal of health counseling may have been provided in the acute care hospital, it is usually when the patient returns home that he is ready to absorb and utilize that information. This provides the rationale for another major responsibility of the medical and nursing services, namely, to educate the patient and his family. Generally, patients are anxious to know about their bodies, what caused the illness, how it will affect their daily living, and how to protect themselves from future problems. In keeping with the overall goals of rehabilitation that are to assist the individual to be as functional as possible and to adjust to his limitations, it is important to teach the patient and his family how to utilize the health care resources available in his community.

## MEDICAL STAFF

While the patient is in the day hospital program, his personal physician should continue to provide primary medical care and prescribe his medical treatment regimen. However, the day hospital is a health facility and, as such, provides medical services to its patients under the direction of the day hospital physician. These medical services should augment, not duplicate, those given by the primary physician. The day hospital physician, who also acts in a consulting role to the primary physician, should be available daily to respond to both minor and major problems of patients. The day hospital should have access to consulting physicians such as cardiologists, internists, neurologists, ophthalmologists, podiatrists, psychiatrists, urologists, dermatologists, and dentists. However, one physician in the day hospital should be designated as medical director and assume responsibility for all medical services provided within the program. The rehabilitation treatment regimen should be under the direction and supervision of a board certified physiatrist. Services usually received by day hospital patients are shown in Appendix M.

### Responsibilities

The medical staff is responsible for defining the medical condition of all patients upon admission and throughout their participation in the program, formulating and implementing medical standards and policies, and for approval of any rehabilitation treatment before it is initiated by the therapist. All patients are given physical examinations upon admission. The extent and degree of examination is determined largely by the amount, kind, and recentness of information that has been provided by the patient's primary physician. If the patient has just been released from an acute hospital where he has undergone extensive diagnostic evaluation, it is neither prudent nor necessary to do another extensive evaluation. Instead, the examining day hospital physician would probably validate the findings of that evaluation. In addition to the physical examination, the day hospital physician should establish what baseline laboratory and other diagnostic data should be performed on admission. For example, he or she would determine whether all patients should have an EKG or only those with known cardiac disease or those who have not had an EKG in the last three months.

In order to satisfy the requirements of regulatory agencies, participants in a day hospital rehabilitation program must be reevaluated monthly by the day hospital physician. At that time, the patient's status and need for continued service must be documented. It must be recognized, however, that patients' medical conditions may, and often do, change from day to day. In a day hospital, medical and nursing staff are dealing with a group of individuals whose underlying health problems affect many organs and systems of the body. In one day hospital, for example, 70 percent of participants had diseases affecting their cardiovascular systems, and nearly all participants had more than one illness; in fact, most health histories revealed three or four major disease categories for each participant. It is therefore recommended that a physician be available for some portion of each day while the program is in session. Many participants will need to be seen more frequently than once a month, and the need for emergency coverage should not be overlooked.

## EMERGENCY CARE

Emergency procedures and equipment should be the same as that used by the parent institution. All medical and nursing personnel, and as many other staff as possible, should be trained in cardiopulmonary resuscitation. Since a physician may not always be readily available, procedures to be followed by other personnel while awaiting his arrival should be formulated and practiced periodically by the staff. There must be written policies and procedures to permit the transfer of the patient in an emergency situation to a nearby acute medical facility. Affiliation agreements must be made with acute care facilities, and arrangements must be made for emergency transportation. It is preferable to transfer a patient to the acute care hospital where his own physician is a member of the attending staff. However, sometimes the patient's condition will not permit this, and a nearby hospital will be the only option.

## NURSING SERVICE

The educational preparation of nurse practitioners and clinical specialists make them the ideal choice for nursing staff in a day hospital. There are three major areas of responsibility of the nurse. These are: (1) comprehensive health assessment and ongoing surveillance of the physical status of patients; (2) health counseling and education of patients, families, and other staff; and (3) coordination of patient care.

### Assessment

The day hospital setting offers a unique opportunity for close collaboration between physician and nurse. Nurses assume responsibility for the preadmission interview, at which time they review the medical data provided by the applicant's personal physician, obtain a health history, and try to ascertain his level of function. The information obtained is measured against the admission criteria to determine eligibility. On the day of admission, the patient is first seen by the nurse who completes the health assessment including a physical examination. The findings are reviewed by the day hospital physician, who also examines the patient, defines the medical problems, clarifies diagnostic questions, orders the specific treatments to ensure proper medical surveillance while the patient is in the program, and validates the need for service.

Protocols developed by the medical and nursing staffs should define the responsibility the day hospital will assume in the medical management of patients. Protocols should consist of a statement of policy and outline the procedures to be followed to ensure implementation of the policy. A sample protocol for diabetes mellitus is provided in Appendix N. Other samples appear in Appendix O. If the protocols are formulated by disease entity or problem classification, they can easily be used in medical and nursing audits to demonstrate quality assurance.

It is important that physicians in the community who have referred patients for rehabilitation be aware of the limits of responsibility that the day hospital is willing to assume in the medical management of their patients. This information may be transmitted in written communication when the patient is accepted into the program or may simply be explained over the telephone.

### Teaching

Teaching or patient education is a nursing responsibility in any setting, but, as was mentioned previously, at the time of admission to a day hospital patients may need more information to be responsive to education. Patients may be enrolled in a day hospital for three or more months, allowing ample time to assess their and their families' need for health education, and then to provide the service. The time factor also affords patients the opportunity to test out their new knowledge in their own home environment and to evaluate their own needs for additional information or practice. The day hospital should provide specific educational programs to meet the individual needs of patients, but it should also recognize the opportunity to provide general information about health. For example, health education classes can be organized around topics such as cancer detection, risk factors in heart disease, nutrition, and medication.

The nursing staff should also play a major role in in-service programs designed for all levels of staff in the day hospital. The health status of participants plays a major role in whether or not they can be rehabilitated. It is important that all staff social workers, physical therapists, occupational therapists, aides, and others understand the physical limitations with which the patient must contend. Patients will be with a staff member every moment that they are in program, and everyone can be trained to assist the nurses in their ongoing assessment of the patient's status.

### Coordination

In order for patients to achieve an improved functional level within their home environment and the community, all staff must work as a team. The success of a team can be enhanced if their efforts on behalf of the patients are skillfully coordinated, and this is dependent on effective communication. The persons best equipped to fulfill this role of coordination are the nurses. They spend a significant amount of time during the day with the patients and have the opportunity to observe them in their therapeutic activities. Their medical knowledge enables them to make professional judgments based on these observations and to communicate significant findings to the appropriate physician. They are also in a position to maintain a dialogue with the families and to evaluate the effects of treatment in the home situation as reported by them. In effect, the nurses serve as catalysts in the patient treatment process.

### Standards of Nursing Practice

Among the many other functions that nurses will perform in the day hospital are skilled nursing procedures. Those procedures include, but are not limited to, insertion of catheters, administration of enemas, care of ostomies, aseptic dressing changes, and the administration of medications. The nursing staff should be prepared to perform whatever technical procedures the patients require while they are participants in the program.

In order for the nursing staff to fulfill this role and assume the other responsibilities that have been discussed, a high degree of skill and competence is required. The following is a summary of the knowledge and skills the nursing staff in a day hospital must possess:

### A.   Knowledge

1.   knowledge of nursing, scientific facts and principles, to enable the nurse to recall and apply relevant knowledge in executing nursing care;
2.   recognition of gaps in knowledge and the ability to locate and utilize appropriate resource material and personnel;
3.   knowledge of symptomatology of major illness categories and the ability to relate these to underlying causes and to follow through with appropriate nursing action;
4.   knowledge of the dynamics of interpersonal relationships and sufficient experience with clients to develop ease and confidence in nursing abilities;
5.   knowledge of the principles of organization and management to enable the nurse to plan, organize, coordinate, and assess the plan of care for a designated caseload;
6.   knowledge of communication skills to enable the nurse to relate effectively to other professional personnel in the delivery of patient care;
7.   knowledge of legal limitations defined in the nurse practice act.

### B.   Management Skills

1.   ability to set priorities with consideration for the availability of time, personnel, and materials, and to be flexible within the framework of day hospital procedures;
2.   demonstrated competence in taking a health history and in recording the history chronologically and succinctly;
3.   ability to utilize the nursing process and to apply its principles to the planning and implementation of specific therapeutic modalities;

4.    ability to monitor and coordinate the client's therapeutic program in a professional manner;

5.    ability to participate effectively in the evaluation of the health plan, to redirect its focus if necessary, and to evaluate its outcome.

### C.   Therapeutic Skills

1.    demonstrated competence in physical assessment, including the techniques of inspection, palpation, percussion, and auscultation, in collaboration with the physician in charge;

2.    ability to examine and review the medication regimen of each client and to assess its efficacy;

3.    competence to meet emergency situations through CPR techniques, hemostasis, first aid for falls and trauma, and knowledge of limitations;

4.    awareness of day hospital procedures regarding emergency treatment and/or transfer of client to acute care;

5.    management of specific devices, such as braces, slings, walkers, and prosthetic devices, and proper techniques in transfers and ambulation.

### D.   Procedural Skills

1.    measurement and interpretation of vital signs.

2.    ability to order and/or carry out diagnostic procedures and tests.

3.    ability to collect specimens for laboratory examinations properly.

### E.   Counseling Skills

1.    sufficient knowledge of the counseling process, as it applies to clients and their families.

2.    ability to organize data and information relevant to the counseling situation.

3.    maturity to assist clients and families in making choices, and to incorporate those choices into the care plan.

**F.   Educational Skills**

1.   ability to teach and direct, as needed, other members of the
     nursing service.
2.   ability to recognize limits of knowledge and experience of
     nursing assistants, and to thoughtfully direct them in attaining
     new knowledge and wider experience.
3.   ability to recognize need for teaching, as opposed to counseling,
     in client's needs for health information.

JOYCE VITALE and BARBARA BERK

## CHAPTER EIGHT

# Speech and Language Therapy

### PROGRAM

Unlike conventional outpatient speech and language clinics for adults, a day hospital speech program is unique in the following respects:

1.  Patients with a speech and/or language pathology participate in a full-day rehabilitation program that reduces physical isolation and provides a setting in which they may socialize with individuals having no communication problems.
2.  It is a comprehensive speech/language program where speech objectives initiated during individual therapy are reinforced in group speech/language therapy and integrated into the total program that includes medical and nursing care, physical therapy, occupational therapy, social service, recreational therapy, midday meal, and transportation. This offers an abundance of opportunities for language stimulation.

Upon admission, all patients whose communication abilities are questionable are referred to the speech department to determine their need and candidacy for speech and language therapy. The majority of these patients suffer from varying degrees of aphasia. A significant number also experience communication problems from inadequate voice and deviant articulation patterns due to neurological disease, trauma, and stroke.

Routine hearing screenings of all patients who have been admitted to the day hospital program are conducted. Those patients whose audiograms indicate inadequate hearing for communication purposes are discussed by the clinical team. If further audiological evaluation is thought to be appropriate, the patient, patient's family, and family physician are consulted concerning a referral to an audiologist for such evaluation.

Once it is determined that speech and/or language therapy is indicated, the patient is placed on a scheduled speech-language program. An extensive evaluation is conducted, if needed. Standardized tests are administered, such as Eisenson's *Examining for Aphasia*, Schuell's *Minnesota Test for Differential Diagnosis*, or the *Porch Index of Communication Abilities* in cases of aphasia. Additional tests administered can be the *Peabody Picture Vocabulary Test*, *The Token Test*, and various articulation tests.

There are varied types of speech and language therapy within the day hospital setting. There is the classic individual therapy, which may be scheduled as needed depending upon the number of days attended; most patients, for example, take part in the program two or three days a week.

Different types of speech/language groups are also part of the program offered. Patients are scheduled for a variety of groups according to individual needs. The groups include:

1.  reading/writing groups;
2.  voice groups;
3.  articulation groups;
4.  homogeneous structured conversation groups;
5.  language-based role-playing groups;
6.  heterogeneous conversation groups.

By using groups in addition to individual therapy, the amount of language output increases. The groups give the patients psychological support. They enhance a patient's realization that he is not alone, that others experience the same difficulties and they, too, are working toward similar goals. This awareness frequently reduces anxiety and enables a patient to work more easily individually. Reinforcement of the skills learned in individual therapy is a major advantage of group therapy. The patient is given yet another chance to practice what he is learning under professional supervision. The reading-writing groups have an additional side benefit. The clinician does not have to spend as much time as might otherwise be required on specific reading-writing skills during the individual therapy sessions; this is done in the groups. If any specific difficulties are noted in a group setting, they can be worked on when a patient is seen individually by the clinician. Reading-writing groups are completely individualized, small in size, averaging four patients, and lasting for periods of approximately 30 minutes. Each person works at his own pace.

Other groups are organized homogeneously according to the degree of language impairment. These groups offer dysphasics a chance to practice the use of functional language with each other within a structured setting. They can also be utilized to stimulate language-based role-playing situations. Patients can, for example, be given opportunities to practice telephoning or shopping. They first practice with each other. Later, once they are comfortable in a simulated setting, they may attempt it in a real-life setting. This takes place only after careful planning by the speech clinician with a family member, a social worker, or possibly a volunteer who would be the supportive influence during the experience. In some cases, the speech pathologist plans and carries out the activity.

### PHYSICAL LAYOUT AND EQUIPMENT

The day hospital clinical area is important. Different types of therapies should be located either in adjoining rooms or within a short distance of each other. This allows patients who may be aided in locomotion by cane, walker, or wheelchair to be able to go from one therapy to the next independently. This accessibility benefits both patients and the clinicians. If patients feel the need to communicate with their clinicians, they can seek them out easily. Clinicians working in this environment benefit from the proximity of the various therapies. They are able to see their patients in unstructured, spontaneous situations, stopping and visiting informally for a few moments. During that time, they can accomplish a number of different things. First, there can be further reinforcement of any language worked on with patients during an individual session. For instance, skills in greeting can be reinforced with a patient who is completely devoid of expressive language. Or a brief, simple conversation can be carried on with a patient who is learning phrases or syntactically correct language, which also reinforces therapy and acts as a reminder that language learned in therapy can be carried over to the real world outside the therapy room. This informality of meetings also enables clinicians to maintain a constant awareness of the progress of current patients and the level of language maintenance of those patients who have been discharged from therapy because they have reached a plateau or achieved the language goals established. This also allows for control of language stimulation during other activities.

The physical set-up necessary for the department of speech services should include the following:

1. individual room for each clinician working on the same day;
2. therapy room for individual and group therapy (small groups of approximately 2 to 3 patients):
   a. desk and possibly a table; a table is necessary if patients cannot use the desk for writing purposes;
   b. blackboard;
   c. mirror;
   d. file cabinet;
   e. bookcase and/or closet to store materials and equipment;
3. therapy room for large group activities (more than 3 or 4 patients):
   a. large table;
   b. cabinet to store materials and supplies.

Diagnostic and evaluation materials that would be necessary to purchase in order to initiate this type of program include:

1. examples of diagnostic and evaluation materials:
   a. Minnesota Test for Differential Diagnosis of Aphasia;
   b. Porch Index of Communicative Ability;
   c. Peabody Picture Vocabulary Test;
   d. Token Test;
   e. Voice Articulation Forms;
   f. Articulation Test;
2. tape recorder;
3. language master—a programmed teaching and reinforcing device;
4. audiometer (if hearing screenings are to be conducted);
5. assorted materials for therapy, including:
   a. matching tasks for objects, colors, forms, and combinations of the latter;
   b. simple, clear pictures of various categories, body parts,

food, beverages, clothing, common objects, rooms, various
modes of transportation;

c. tasks for the purpose of working on concrete and abstract
language concepts;

d. materials for reading:
(1) printed words for the purpose of matching word to
picture and/or object;
(2) simple reading comprehension exercises;
(3) books, appropriate for adults, beginning on Grade I
level;
(4) magazines appropriate for adults;

e. materials for writing, including exercises for:
(1) copying;
(2) spelling;
(3) writing of simple sentences;
(4) writing of letters, paragraphs, and so forth;

f. development of materials by speech pathologist:
(1) a screening instrument to ascertain quickly the
need for speech/language therapy;
(2) an evaluation flow sheet, comprised of a breakdown
of all modalities based on a five-point scale and
indicating speech/language proficiency, to enable
other disciplines to interpret a patient's speech/
language level and compare a patient's status from
evaluation to reevaluation;
(3) pictures of familiar objects for use in individual and
group therapy, as well as for homework or to reinforce
language learned.

## INTERDISCIPLINARY TEAM APPROACH

The team approach at the day hospital is actually that: each
department has its own individuality, but the major focus is the
patient and helping him to achieve his functional goals. Because of
this interest and the integration of the various therapy teams and
nursing staff, the patient benefits fully. Interdepartmental competition is reduced to a minimum. Each staff member is fully aware
of the benefit to the patient from participation in a total integrated
program. Thus, full support is given by all to his speech and language
attempts. This integrative, multidisciplinary approach enables  the

speech pathologist to train professional and paraprofessional, paid personnel and students to comprehend and deal with speech/language patients.

Day hospital staff continually communicate with each other concerning the status of the patients. Once again, the physical design plays an important role. The clinician is able to discuss informally a patient's communicative abilities with all members of the staff and demonstrate to other staff members who also work with the patient just how and what language to reinforce. Most often, this is done quite casually while patients are involved in an activity or moving from one therapy to another. It is not necessary to wait for a formal in-service program. The clinician can also observe informally whether what should be reinforced is actually accomplished or is presented correctly to the patient. This staff reinforcement is a great aid in a patient's language acquisition because it offers an immediate positive response to his language attempts.

Frequent in-service conferences are held with the nursing and therapy assistants to discuss the patients and to improve the understanding and support they are providing. During these conferences, ways of promoting language acquisition are discussed and stressed.

### STAFFING

Of a total day hospital population, it is estimated that one quarter to one third of the patients will exhibit dysfunction in the areas of speech and language. One full-time speech pathologist would be needed for each 35 to 40 patients per day. This is based on the following:

1.  a total caseload of 12 or 13 patients a day;
2.  half-hour sessions for both individual and group therapy from 9 a.m. through 3 p.m., with the two remaining hours allotted for administrative purposes, family counseling, meetings, reports, and evaluations.

Volunteers can be used in the speech and language program. They are taught what language area a patient is working on, and they offer patients yet another chance for reinforcement. The volunteers are trained and supervised closely by the speech clinician. Volunteers are also utilized to lead discussion groups with high-level dysphasic patients. They can lead groups on current events or stimulate conversation during informal gatherings, for example, when patients are preparing to go home or are having refreshments.

Volunteers working in other departments are often in close contact with the speech pathologist. The social worker, for example, attempts to get the patient involved in the community. When the patient also has communication problems, both departments work together to get the patient ready for these new experiences. A volunteer may go into the home or take the patient out shopping on a day the patient does not attend the day hospital.

### FAMILY INVOLVEMENT

Since day hospital patients go home every night and very often attend the day hospital only two or three times a week, the family is an extremely important source of support and reinforcement. Quite often family members are pessimistic and discouraged when dealing with individuals who are extremely deficient in language. However, if the clinician demonstrates ways in which the patient will be able to perform with some success, the family is encouraged and more willing to help. The family is very much in need of a ray of hope and of positive professional support; the speech clinician provides some of this.

Family members and/or attendants are usually willing to come into the day hospital to learn how to reinforce and handle a patient's language level. As noted in one type of group therapy, the family (usually a spouse) often can furnish the structured situation an aphasic patient needs when he is first attempting speech situations outside the protection of home and hospital.

RENEE SCHLESINGER

*CHAPTER NINE*

# *Physical Therapy*

## PROGRAM

Physical therapy in the day hospital is concerned with the treatment of people with a disability caused by disease or injury. It consists of a planned program to relieve symptoms, improve function, and prevent further disability.

The physical therapist, in consultation with the multidisciplinary rehabilitation team including the day hospital physician, will develop a treatment program, setting realistic goals to meet each patient's special needs. These needs will be determined after a thorough evaluation by each member of the treatment team to ascertain the patient's physical status and functional ability. Not only will the patient's disabilities be considered, but also his abilities. The physical therapist, as a member of the multidisciplinary rehabilitation team, will help meet not only the physical, but also the emotional and social needs of each patient. Continuous assessment will be necessary as the patient gradually recovers, so that his returning abilities can be as useful as possible.

The treatment plan may be carried out during individual sessions or in group activities.

Physical therapy includes:

A. evaluation;
B. therapeutic exercise;

C.  modalities;
D.  massage;
E.  ambulation training;
F.  family conferences;
G.  home visits.

The following is a description of each of these components of a physical therapy program.

### A.  Evaluation

The evaluation of a patient by a physical therapist usually requires 30 minutes to one hour on a one-to-one basis. In some cases, if verbal communication is not possible, additional time may be spent in gaining information from the person accompanying the patient. Both physical and functional status should be evaluated with an evaluatory tool to be used throughout his stay at the day hospital to measure progress. After the initial evaluation, problems are determined, goals set, and length of stay estimated in cooperation with the treatment team. This should all be discussed both with the patient and with the family.

### B.  Therapeutic Exercise

This treatment may range from 30 to 60 minutes, depending on the needs of the patient and his individual endurance. It may be carried out in combination with other treatments such as modalities, massage, or ambulation training. Various types of exercise may be done to improve strength, endurance, coordination, range of motion and mobility, and to decrease pain.

Exercises may include various facilitation techniques for both relaxation and strengthening. Therapeutic exercise may also include the teaching and practice of functional activities such as moving about in bed, transfers, and rising from a chair. Although the patient may and should be taught exercises to be done independently at home, he responds best and is motivated by an individually addressed request for movement. In addition to these individual exercises, a patient may benefit from independent activities such as use of a stationary bicycle or restorator, work on overhead pulleys, or weight lifting.

Therapeutic exercise may also be pursued in a group. This could be a completely separate session lasting one hour. Part of the time is spent in arranging the group, transferring patients to chairs, and handing out equipment. These exercises provide motivation and socialization as well as mobility. The group should consist of patients at similar levels of ability. Some mobility games, such as ball playing or bean bag throwing, may be added to the program for this group. This kind of activity could also be done as diversional program to implement the patient's therapeutic exercise.

### C.   Modalities

A modality may be given singly or in combination. A treatment session done alone usually lasts 30 minutes, but is more often done in combination with massage and/or therapeutic exercise. Modalities used at the day hospital might be hydrocolator packs, paraffin, diathermy, ultrasound, cold packs, traction, electrical stimulation, or TENS (transcutaneous electrical nerve stimulator). These would be used to relieve pain and relax a person for preparation for exercise and functional activity. Biofeedback may also be used for relaxation or muscle reeducation.

### D.   Massage

A massage session usually lasts for 10 to 15 minutes, but almost always would be done in combination with application of heat.

### E.   Ambulation Training

Ambulation training may take from 15 minutes to one hour, depending on each patient's tolerance. It is often carried out in combination with exercise. It might be beneficial in many cases to pursue ambulation training several times a day. This can be done by all staff in a day hospital setting. Depending on the patient's abilities, a therapist might begin teaching independent wheelchair propulsion and then progress, as tolerated, to walking inside or outside parallel hemi bars, with or without ambulation aids. The amount of supervision a patient requires during ambulation should be determined, and this information should be available to all members of the rehabilitation team to enable the patient to be walking as much as possible with maximum safety. A fall could be catastrophic to the rehabilitation program and to the patient's confidence. Once a patient walks well on level surfaces, he may progress to stair climbing, ramp climbing, walking outdoors on all surfaces, learning to manage a curb or bus step, and getting up from the floor.

Ambulation training may include the assessment and/or prescription of a prosthetic or orthotic device. This should be done in consultation with the day hospital physician and orthotist/prosthetist.

### F.    Family Conferences

It is important to instruct the patient and his family, friends, or homemaker in the use of appliances, therapeutic exercises, and anything else that will make the patient's life at the day hospital and at home more comfortable. It is the aim to help him to achieve and maintain his maximum function. A home exercise program should be written out and taught both to patient and to family. The capabilities of the patient should be known by the family so that they may help the patient when necessary but enable him to do what he is capable of himself. It is often more difficult to stand by and allow a loved one to struggle. The physical therapist should be available to answer questions both of the patient and of the family.

### G.    Home Visits

In some cases a home visit may be beneficial, probably in the company of the occupational therapist, to assess most effectively the needs of the patient at home. Equipment may be required or alterations made to the home. It might benefit the patient to practice stair climbing with the therapist in the home setting. A written report with recommendations should follow the home visit. The appropriate member of the treatment team can then practice or work out the patient's problems while he is still at the day hospital.

### PHYSICAL LAYOUT AND EQUIPMENT

The organization of a physical therapy department with two large, connecting rooms works out well. One room, which is used for individual clinic sessions and ambulation training, should be set up with treatment mats and curtain dividers for privacy. It can also contain parallel bars and practice stairs, which are helpful for ambulation training. The other room is used for group exercises, with sturdy chairs available for all patients. This could also be available for ambulation of patients and other activities when not being used for group sessions.

The size of the rooms depends on the number and type of patients being treated. A treatment cubicle requires a space of at least 8' X 10'; one set of parallel bars also requires at least 8' X 10'. There must be room for a staff office, linen, and storing of supplies and equipment.

A basic list of equipment includes:

1. several plinths, including some low mats and some regular-height or adjustable-height treatment tables;
2. hydrocolator pack machine with hydrocolator packs and covers;
3. paraffin machine;
4. several masonite boards to be used as powder boards for gravity and eliminated exercise;
5. several sturdy chairs with and without arms;
6. graded velcro weights 1 to 10 lbs;
7. push-up blocks;
8. quadriceps board;
9. a goniometer;
10. cold pack machine;
11. ultrasound;
12. traction unit;
13. overhead pulleys;
14. a cabinet for storing equipment;
15. other physical therapy modalities would depend on the needs of the particular department, but might include diathermy, electrical stimulation, TENS, and biofeedback;
16. restorators;
17. parallel bars;
18. hemi bar;
19. stairs with curb and bus step;
20. assorted canes and walkers and tips;
21. adjustable slings;
22. assorted braces with shoes to be used for practice;
23. wands;
24. various games—bean bags, balls;
25. music to be used for group activities.

Hydrotherapy might be helpful for many day hospital patients, but would require additional staffing and space.

There are also indirect patient services that must be accounted for when planning a day hospital physical therapy department, such as the recording of progress notes or of attendance. In-service education and meetings and conferences must be considered. The maintenance of the equipment and department is also important.

### STAFFING

The staffing pattern depends on the number of patients and the particular type of patient being treated. A physical therapy department must be under the supervision of a registered physical therapist. The direct patient care is carried out by a registered physical therapist. A physical therapy assistant and/or aide may assume some responsibilities under the direct supervision of a registered physical therapist.

NANCY BENES

## CHAPTER TEN

# *Occupational Therapy and Therapeutic Activities*

### PROGRAM

Occupational therapy is a planned program to improve function, to prevent further disability, and/or to assist the patient in adjusting to residual function. The unique feature of occupational therapy is in the use of activities to achieve the ultimate goal of optimum patient functioning. Exercise modalities may be used to increase the patient's physical abilities for use in purposeful activity.

The occupational therapy department in the day hospital should be set up to include:

A.　functional exercises;
B.　functional activities;
C.　activities of daily living;
D.　homemaking;
E.　perceptual training;
F.　communications—socialization;
G.　evaluation of equipment needs;
H.　home visits and evaluation;
I.　group therapeutic activities.

In planning an occupational therapy program, each of the above categories should be clearly outlined as to purpose and what the activity might include.

The following are examples of activities that might be included in each of the suggested program components:

### A. Functional Exercises

1.  the use of counterbalance slings to improve the range of motion and strength of the shoulder and shoulder girdle;
2.  the ball-bearing exercise skate-board, the inclined board, the powder board, the pseudosanders (with and without resistance), used to improve the range of motion of the shoulder, elbow, and wrist, as well as finger strengthening and grasp;
3.  stacking and unstacking cardboard cones, used to promote range of motion against gravity;
4.  arranging and placing small wooden cubes or plastic pegs in a design to achieve fine-finger dexterity, grasp, and coordination;
5.  theraplast exercises to improve individual finger and overall hand strength.

### B. Functional Activities

These may include any craft that enables the patient to engage in active, nonstatic exercise, with built-in elements of repetition, range of motion, resistance, and coordination of affected joints and muscles. For example, woodworking is used in a variety of ways, according to the requirements of the individual patient. It provides action rather than maintained contraction, except for the finger flexion needed for holding tools. It aids in developing grasp. Sawing and sanding of wood provide repetition of motion and can be graduated in difficulty for range of motion, resistance, and coordination exercises.

### C. Activities of Daily Living or Self-Care Ability

Based upon assessment of existing capacity, patients are taught self-feeding, grooming, bathing, dressing, communications, and bed and wheelchair transfers. Activities may involve training in holding down paper while writing, filling a coffee cup, use of telephone.

As the patients's needs dictate, special one-handed devices, such as a long-handled shoehorn or sponge, button-aide, zipper pull, reachers, and rocker knives are used to increase the patient's independence.

### D.   Homemaking

Needs are assessed and goals formulated consistent with the physical capacities of the patient. Duties required in maintaining a household, namely, cleaning, cooking, bed making, laundry, and shopping are included. For example, if cooking skills need improvement, special recipes or dishes are used to provide practice in mixing, chopping, cutting, peeling, pouring, measuring, and using surface burners and ovens.

### E.   Perceptual Training

This involves assessment and training of a patient to be able to give meaning to what he sees and to help him to integrate past visual experiences with those presently seen. It may include coordinated movements of eye and hand (visual motor); visual recognition of forms and figures against increasingly complex grounds (figure ground relationships); perception of shape, size, color, texture, and position in space of geometric figures (constancy of shape); and training in increasing the patient's ability to visually relate his body in relation to other objects and people, or objects in relation to other objects (spatial relationships).

Perceptual training encourages the patient to compensate in those tasks that are important to him. It helps the patient to:

1.   judge distances more accurately when performing a transfer, wheeling his chair, or walking into other objects;
2.   not to disregard the affected side of his body and to be more aware of crossing the midline;
3.   to be able to carry out tasks such as dressing or preparing a meal by a breakdown of each task, using short, direct verbal cues to meet the needs of the individual;
4.   to utilize aids to compensate for loss, such as using a ruler or a specially cut card to structure material being read.

### F. Communications and Socialization

Loss of communication skills causes intense frustration. Occupational therapy reinforces speech therapy by providing stimulation and support, which encourages the patient to participate in verbal communication. The patient is also encouraged to relearn handwriting and typewriting skills.

### G. Evaluation of Equipment Needs

Special equipment may be constructed within the occupational therapy department to be used by patients at home in order to increase their functional independence, such as transfer board for use in the bathtub. Equipment needs should be evaluated and equipment ordered or provided.

### H. Home Visits and Evaluation

An occupational therapist can be available to make on-the-site visits to the homes of individual patients, at the request of the treatment team. At this time, an evaluation of the home setting can be made to determine areas of household proficiency and/or limitation of the patient. Emphasis is placed on work simplification techniques, such as:

arranging work areas within normal reach or within easy reach of a wheelchair;

sliding objects rather than lifting or carrying them by using a wheelchair lapboard or rolling table;

stabilization of kitchen tools and appliances;

selection of tools which require only one hand to operate;

negotiation of barriers that thwart independence, such as too narrow halls and doorways, door sills, or entrance steps, where these cannot be eliminated;

finding solutions to additional problems involving placement of electrical outlets and switches, inaccessible closets, and poor furniture arrangements allowing little maneuvering space;

and the possible relocation or replanning of rooms
and/or adding a bathroom on the first floor of the home.

A written report with recommendations is made upon completion
of the home visit to become a part of the patient's treatment plan
and permanent medical record. Assessment of necessary changes
should be correlated with the individual patient's performance in
homemaking training and in activities of daily living. Additional
training can be given to the patient, if deemed necessary, while the
patient is still being treated in the day hospital. Equipment and
devices may also be ordered at this time and arrangements made for
installation of grab bars, extended showers, or toilet safety rails.

### I.   Group Therapeutic Activities

A planned program consisting of structured crafts, creative
crafts, manual crafts, games, community service projects, patient
news publications, and group homemaking can meet the needs of
those patients who do not require individual therapy, but who have
deficits that would be improved by participation in a group setting.
Patients should not be maintained in this program for diversional
reasons, but should have a clearly defined reason (obtainable goal)
for being there.

1.  The structured craft program is designed to incorporate one
    or more of the following goals:
    a.   improvement of coordination and/or prevention of deterio-
         ration;
    b.   improvement in range of motion and/or prevention of loss
         of range of motion;
    c.   improvement in strength in upper extremities to facilitate
         independence in self-care activities;
    d.   improvement of perceptual skills;
    e.   increase of endurance through graded activities;
    f.   improvement in cognitive functioning by including activities
         graded in terms of complexity, orientation activities, and
         varied degrees of instruction aimed at increasing indepen-
         dence;
    g.   improvement in communication skills in cooperation with
         speech therapy, including writing, typing, letter- and word-
         oriented activities.
2.  The manual craft program is designed to incorporate one or
    more of the following goals and to provide:

  a.  heavy resistive activities for strengthening or improving function of the upper extremities;
  b.  increase in range of motion through elevated activities;
  c.  fine finger coordination activities by assembling projects;
  d.  simple repetitive projects for patients incapable of following through with projects requiring more than automatic response;
  e.  promotion of avocational interests for possible carry-over in the home.

3.  The creative crafts program is designed to stimulate the patient's interest level and creativity in a nonstructured medium. This program:
  a.  is an area of activity that is not necessarily planned to meet the physical needs of the patients, but to offer a stimulating, satisfying craft program that directs attention to the emotional, social, and creative needs of the patient;
  b.  provides an educational avenue where reality orientation can be expanded and the patient's self-esteem increased through mastery of crafts;
  c.  allows for mental stimulation by motivating patients to follow instructions, to make decisions, and to learn new skills;
  d.  gives opportunities for socialization of patients by sharing in similar projects and contributing their ideas and experiences within the relaxed atmosphere of varied craft and art media.

4.  Games are planned activities structured to meet one or more of the following goals:
  a.  reality orientation through games of awareness: to make patients aware or keep them aware of time, place, and person;
  b.  remotivation through games of challenge: to provide opportunities for expression of imagination, creativity, and for mental stimulation;
  c.  socialization through games of encounter with others: to provide enrichment of life through interpersonal relationships, positive use of leisure time and relaxation.
  d.  general physical conditioning through games of action and agility: to provide exercise to improve or prevent physical deterioration.
  e.  cognitive integration through games of personal enrichment.
  Noncraft/game activities can be added as the program develops and patient needs become clearer.

5.  Community service projects are designed as outreach groups to

alert patients to the needs of others in the community, to make them more aware of resources available to them, and to prepare patients for discharge through group support.

6.   Patient news publications are structured to meet the needs of the patient requiring more intellectual stimulation, for patients needing an avenue to increase communications skills, and for those who are unable to participate on a physical level in other activities.

7.   Group homemaking is intended to provide, in a relaxed group atmosphere, opportunities to perfect previously acquired skills or new techniques, build confidence through doing, share in problem-solving, and to encourage diet awareness.

Patients should be assessed by the occupational therapy department on the first day of admission. A plan of care should be written up including evaluation of deficits and obtainable goals. Total staff should also confer on their individual goals and outline a total treatment plan for the patient. Patients should be reevaluated periodically.

As patients progress toward meeting goals, some individuals may graduate to a program of therapeutic activities where groups of patients are seen under the supervision of a registered occupational therapist. They are scheduled for specific activities according to their needs for continued therapy, their skills, and their interests. These groups can be led by paraprofessional, in-service trained staff.

An occupational therapy treatment may consist of one-half hour to 50 minutes of patient participation in one or more treatment modalities, depending upon the individual patient's needs, fatigability, and endurance.


### PHYSICAL LAYOUT AND EQUIPMENT

The following are the basic equipment and space needs for an occupational therapy department in a day hospital for 35 to 40 patients:


I.   Occupational Therapy Clinic Area

A.   *Physical setup:*

1.   large room, approximately 23' X 30';
2.   four large round tables, 4' diameter;

3. twenty strong, light-weight armchairs;
4. four straight-backed chairs;
5. three large metal storage cabinets, 3′ × 6′;
6. one utility sink.

B. *Equipment:*

1. three slant-boards with sliding boxes;
2. six pseudosanders;
3. six one-hand mitts;
4. one skate-board;
5. weights: one 5 lbs; five 2½ lbs; five 1¼ lbs;
6. Perceptual Training Equipment:
   a. three large Parquetry and Design Cards;
   b. three colored large Inch Cubes and Design cards;
   c. three peg boards and pegs and boards;
   d. design dominoes;
   e. coins and bills;
   f. coin puzzles;
7. two holders for embroidery and knitting;
8. one footstool;
9. one counterbalance or Deltoid slings;
10. four detachable arm slings;
11. one electric sewing machine;
12. one ironing board;
13. one steam iron;
14. one electric typewriter;
15. two left-handed scissors.

## II. Woodworking and Art Area

A. *Physical setup:*

1. room, approximately 15′ × 24′;
2. one large table, 3′ × 9′ (heavy hardwood);
3. six strong, light-weight armchairs;
4. four large metal storage cabinets, 3′ × 6′;
5. one utility sink;
6. one large, galvanized iron garbage can with tight-fitting cover.

B. *Equipment:*

1. rip saw;
2. cross cut saw;

  3. mitre box;
  4. electric sabre saw;
  5. electric drill and bits;
  6. hand drill and bits;
  7. files, assorted cuts;
  8. screwdrivers, assorted sizes—including one Phillips screw-driver;
  9. C-clamps, 4";
  10. C-clamps, 3";
  11. small table vises;
  12. assortment of nails, brads, and screws;
  13. assortment of sandpaper.


III. **Activities of Daily Living Area (Also used for evaluations)**

A. *Physical setup:*

  1. room, approximately 14' × 14';
  2. one low bed with two pillows;
  3. one bed pull;
  4. one footstool;
  5. one table, 3' × 3';
  6. two chairs;
  7. one commode with removable arms;
  8. one dresser with mirror.

B. *Equipment—self-care devices:*

  1. reachers, assorted;
  2. rocker knife;
  3. long-handled bath sponge;
  4. long-handled comb, toothbrush, fork and spoon;
  5. long-handled shoehorn;
  6. stocking aid;
  7. built-up eating utensils;
  8. plate guard;
  9. elastic shoelaces;
  10. apron hoop;
  11. universal cuff;
  12. cup, spillproof;
  13. foam padding for building up utensils.

C. *Supplies*

  1. velcro, white and black, 1";

2. theraplast;
3. orthoplast.


## IV. Bathroom Area (including bathtub, toilet and sink)

*A. Physical setup:*

1. room, approximately 10′ × 12′;
2. toilet safety rails;
3. hi-rise seat;
4. Homer Higgs bathtub seat;
5. two grab bars near tub;
6. suction tub seat;
7. life guard rail;
8. transfer tub seat;
9. one wooden chair, approximately same height as bathtub;
10. non-skid tape treads;
11. rubber bath mat;
12. showerall;
13. transfer board.


## V. Kitchen Area and Homemaking Area

*A. Physical setup:*

1. room, approximately 15′ × 18′;
2. small kitchen table with two chairs;
3. electric stove;
4. refrigerator;
5. sink;
6. counter space;
7. electric dryer;
8. electric washing machine.

*B. Specialized equipment:*

1. rolling utility table;
2. electric one-handed can opener;
3. wooden bowl holder;
4. electric mixer;
5. wheelchair lapboard;
6. suction nail brush;

7.  spike board for peeling and cutting vegetables;
8.  glass washer brush;
9.  handle stabilizer;
10. wall-hung over-stove mirror;
11. long-handled wooden spoons;
12. grater holder;
13. Zim jar lid opener;
14. flip-top garbage can;
15. dish drainer and rubber mat;
16. long-handled dust pan and broom;
17. walker basket, adjustable;
18. wet mop.


VI.  **Storage Area**

A.  *Physical setup:*

1.  room, approximately 11' X 14';
2.  shelving.

B.  *Supplies:*

Scissors, tile, assorted sizes and colors; metal bases; tile cutters;
white glue; glue containers; leather tools; flame resistant lace;
leather kits; copper; repousse tools; escutcheon pins; plastelene;
liver of sulphur; silicone spray; poppit beads; golf tees; wood
projects (pre-cut); no-frame rug canvas; latch needles; Turkish
Knot weaving looms; cotton warp; fabric; twine; Cotton Roving;
rug yarn; Peacock loom; sewing thread; sewing machine needles;
plastic baskets; varnish; paints; shellac; thinner; alcohol; paint
brushes; plywood; lumber; cardboard cones; masking tape;
needle threaders; papers—construction, water color, drawing,
manila; artists' paints—water color, acrylic, oil, tempera;
colored pencils; charcoal; pastels; rubber cement; clay.


VII. **Evaluation Equipment**

1.  goniometers, small and large;
2.  dynamometer;
3.  peg board;
4.  2D and 3D puzzles;
5.  two test tubes with stoppers.

**VIII. Additional Equipment for Group Therapeutic Activities**

1.  gardening: tools, pots, Gro-light, soil;
2.  music: piano, rhythm instruments, record player;
3.  games: scrabble, board games, checkers, ping-pong table, table shuffleboard;
4.  news publication: collating, duplicating, paper cutting, silk screen equipment, blackboard;
5.  education–recreation: movie screen, slide projector, camera.

**IX. Office Area**

A. *Physical setup:*

1.  two desks with chairs;
2.  one file cabinet;
3.  one bookcase.

**STAFFING**

An occupational therapy department is administered by, or is under the direct supervision of, a registered occupational therapist. The prescribed treatment may be carried out by an occupational therapist, an occupational therapy assistant, or occupational therapy aide.

**DIVERSIONAL ACTIVITIES**

The program components discussed thus far are essentially prescriptive. An additional element that is supportive of the various facets of the occupational therapy program, is more recreational and diversional in nature. While it is not prescriptive, it is, nonetheless structured and purposeful.

The day hospital therapeutic regimen can be taxing for the patients. It is tailored to each patient's needs as specified in the comprehensive assessment. An important part of the regimen calls for interspersing the prescribed activities with those aimed at "distraction," "refreshment," "relaxation." Music and dance are key features of a diversional program. Dancing as it would be used with day hospital patients is motion to music—swaying, tapping of the hands or feet, snapping of the fingers, movement of the hands and/or head—an involvement of the patient with the distraction this activity provides. Observation of patients as they are induced to participate provides evidence of how "the dance" relaxes. Music, in particular, has a special therapeutic and renewing effect. Classical music with a very slow, stately, restful rhythm has been shown to reduce blood pressure, slow the heartbeat, and slow brain waves to an alpha rhythm. Paradoxically, it increases mental alertness; it permits the individual to attend to the environment in a relaxed, nonfatiguing way. To some degree, it has an effect similar to meditation without the accompanying need for training and individual effort.[1]

It is well known that chronically ill, disabled individuals, such as most patients attending a day hospital, have undergone and may be undergoing considerable physical and psychic trauma. This may result in varying levels of somatic preoccupation, with excessive concern for one's health. In part, this self-absorption represents an unconscious regressive retreat toward a more dependent position.[2] Frequently the behavior of the individual in seeking increased attention and gratification of dependency needs succeeds in turning away the persons who can satisfy the needs. Very often a vicious cycle of behavior ensues that interferes with the planned therapeutic efforts. Sometimes the failure to achieve the sought-after gratification results in withdrawal by the individual, followed by virtual isolation. The relaxing effect of appropriate music, with the attendant mental alertness, may interrupt a patient's absorption with self long enough to permit suggestions that could break preoccupation.

Luncheon get-togethers involving preparation, serving, and eating a meal offer an opportunity to help individual patients focus on the needs of fellow patients. Group discussions/seminars on significant current events enlarge the psychosocial world that has been narrowed by disabling illness. Special events such as birthdays, anniversaries, holidays, and visits by community groups offer welcome interruptions in everyday routines. All of these, plus myriad other activities constitute the core of recreational/diversional service. An indispensable part of such a program, however, is professional direction by a thoroughly trained person with a solid grounding in knowledge of human behavior and its wellsprings of motivation. This person should be sensitive, empathic, and skilled in interpersonal relationships. Under the direction of a recreational therapist, well-trained volunteers, carefully chosen for their concern for ill, disabled persons, can carry out a stimulating, innovative, genuinely therapeutic program that will reinforce the other elements of the day hospital treatment.

## NOTES

1. Laughlin, Henry P., *The Ego and Its Defenses* (New York: Appleton-Century-Crofts, 1970).
2. Ostrander, Sheila, and Lynn Schroeder, *Superlearning* (New York: Delacorte Press/Confucian Press, 1979).

JULIANA SNYDER

*CHAPTER ELEVEN*

# *Guidelines for Nutrition Services*

Nutritional guidance for the adult in a day hospital setting is partly a science and partly an art. The challenge for the nutritionist and the other health care team members lies in balancing the two. A nutritionally adequate diet must be planned within any medically indicated restrictions. Consideration must also be given to personal preferences and the cultural background of individual patients. Normally, the patient receives a noon-time meal, plus morning and afternoon refreshments. The other two meals are taken at home where there is no dietary control. For that reason, nutritional counseling and education with patients and family members are significant.

Food service arrangements will vary depending upon the available resources, including budgetary constraints. Food service may be provided directly within the day hospital by day hospital staff. Or, if it is part of a larger institution, the food service department there may prepare and deliver the meals. Some day hospitals make contractual arrangements with community-based nutrition centers or "Meals on Wheels" programs or commercial vendors for delivery of the noontime meal. The following guidelines should be modified to fit the particular situation that is in effect.

## OBJECTIVES

The objectives of a nutrition service are:

1. to serve a nutritious, well-balanced noon meal to patients;
2. to assess the nutritional status of all patients;
3. to provide nutritional counseling and therapeutic diet instruction to all patients, family members, and home health care personnel as deemed necessary by the members of the health team;
4. to provide in-service education for staff members;
5. to provide for snacks, nourishments, and special parties and events, as needed.

### STANDARDS

The standards that must be met for a successful food service operation are the following:

1. There shall be an organized dietetic service, directed by a qualified person and staffed by adequate numbers of dietitians and technical and clerical personnel.
2. The dietetic service shall have adequate space, equipment, and supplies to effect the efficient, safe, and sanitary operation of all functions assigned to it.
3. There shall be written policies and procedures that govern all food service activities.
4. The administration of the nutritional aspects of patient care shall be under the direction of a qualified dietitian.

### FOOD SERVICES ARRANGEMENTS

The following are three possible arrangements for food service in a day hospital:

1. Creation of a food service establishment when none is presently available:
   It is possible to establish a kitchen, hire food service personnel, and prepare a satisfactory noon meal for day hospital patients; however, to do this, all standards, prevailing health laws, and sanitary codes must be followed in order for the kitchen to operate.
   The following steps must be taken:

    a.   hire a food service manager or consultant dietitian to plan and direct the food service;

    b.   plan the kitchen; purchase equipment; establish all policies and procedures;

    c.   adopt a diet manual;

    d.   create an identification system of patient trays and meals;

    e.   employ competent food service workers;

    f.   plan menus;

    g.   order food for preparation;

    h.   train and supervise employees;

    i.   follow all sanitation and safety procedures;

    j.   use disposable dishes if dishwasher is not purchased.

2.    To cater for a noon meal for day hospital patients, the following steps must be taken:

    a.   contact all area food service establishments:

        (1)   restaurants or cafeterias;

        (2)   food service teaching programs, such as vocational schools, chef's colleges, culinary institutes;

        (3)   local institutional food service establishments, such as hospitals, nursing homes, adult homes;

    b.   examine all available food services, and evaluate their capabilities for providing nutritious meals and cost-controlled meal service; a consultant dietitian must assist with this evaluation.

3.    Food service for day hospital as an extension of an existing health care facility (hospital, extended care and health related care facilities, adult homes, and existing nutrition programs):

    It is best to utilize the existing food service in these instances, rather than attempt to establish a separate one.

    The following steps must be taken:

    a.   establish the type of menu desired:

        (1)   selective; or

        (2)   nonselective;

    b.   establish cost per meal;

    c.   arrange for therapeutic diet meals, according to adopted diet manual for diabetic, calorie-restricted, fat-restricted, sodium-restricted, bland, and soft diets;

    d.   discuss and establish a viable method for acquiring needed snacks, supplemental nourishment, and foods for parties or special events; morning coffee break or afternoon juice breaks may be essential, depending on the needs of the patients;

e. establish meal substitutes for patients with food intolerances or dislikes;

f. teach day hospital staff how to serve meals to make meal-time pleasant for the patients and to return the used food service equipment to dietary in an acceptable manner.

### DIETARY COUNSELING

Enforcement of the standard that the administration of the nutritional aspects of patient care shall be under the direction of a qualified dietitian is of great importance in the day hospital situation. Day hospital patients generally consume only the noon meal and snacks in the day hospital setting and then return to their homes and the community at the end of the day. Individuals must, therefore, be able to manage their own nutritional intake and/or special diet, so it is imperative that they receive the necessary information and guidance to do this.

### STAFFING

Employment of a dietitian or nutritionist who is a member of the American Dietetics Association, preferably a registered dietitian, is recommended. An individual with a master's degree and/or experience in the public health field is desirable. A shared position with the present food service dietitian in an institution can also be created, as long as the services listed below can be provided.

### SERVICES AND PROGRAM

The services provided by the nutrition consultant should include, but not necessarily be limited to, the following areas:

1. nutritional assessment, which includes a complete nutritional history from patients and/or reliable family members; evaluation of the patient's nutritional intake; further interviews with the family and patient; periodic reevaluation of the patient's nutritional intake;

2.  instruction in the principles of good nutrition as needed;
3.  individual or group diet counseling aimed at teaching the patient and/or the person preparing his meals the principles of good nutrition and the requirements of a therapeutic diet, if one is ordered;
4.  creation of written policies and procedures for all nutrition services;
5.  staff instruction in nutrition and therapeutic diets provided either individually or through scheduled in-service education classes; the nutrition consultant should recommend suitable library materials and acquire or create a file of workable materials for staff and patients;
6.  noting of significant likes and dislikes or food intolerances that may require substitution at mealtime; dissemination of this information to appropriate personnel and recording in patients' charts.
7.  consultation within the day hospital and with food service concerning appropriate snacks and refreshments, nourishments procedures, methods of ordering patient meals, and meal service within the day hospital; all problems encountered should be communicated to the food service establishment providing meal services;
8.  participation in team meetings and conferences to share nutritional goals with staff from other disciplines and to receive feedback about patients' dietary habits as observed in the course of the day hospital program;
9.  charting of pertinent nutritional information and observations on the patient's medical record;
10. making a diet manual available and seeing that it is utilized within the day hospital.

The number of hours per week that the nutrition consultant is on duty is established by the policy of the day hospital, the number of patients, and the patients' needs.

A workable system of scheduling patients for nutritional consultation should be established in conjunction with the clinical coordinator.

## CHAPTER TWELVE

# Social Work

The primary goal of the social work department in a day hospital is to enhance the physical and social rehabilitation of each individual patient, with particular emphasis on reintegration into community life. Active members of the interdisciplinary team, social workers provide direct services to patients and their families predicated on the belief that comprehensive patient care requires concurrent treatment of psychosocial and physical problems. Each patient admitted to a day hospital should be assigned to a particular social worker who will be responsible for assisting him with pertinent personal problems and any environmental difficulties related to his physical and social rehabilitation. Staff will be dealing with the patient's adjustment to illness and the resulting functional impairments as it relates to the home environment. Of prime importance is consideration of the realities of the patient's situation in determining the base for necessary social service.

## PLANNING AND ORGANIZATION

The social work staff plans, organizes, and coordinates the delivery of social work services as an integral part of health care, and periodically reviews the effectiveness of services rendered. When appropriate, it participates in policy determination and in program planning. It identifies and documents areas for improvement and change, presenting pertinent proposals through appropriate channels.

## ORIENTATION OF PATIENTS AND THEIR FAMILIES

The intake and orientation process is directed toward completing a psychosocial assessment of the patient and facilitating his adjustment to the program. This begins on the first day of the patient's admission. The presenting problems should be identified and social work treatment goals defined and integrated into the overall treatment plan. Telephone and personal discussions should be held with the patient's caretaker (usually a family member) and other collateral sources previously or currently involved in the patient's care. Family members and "significant others" should be seen individually and with the patient, where possible. They should be invited to attend family group workshops. The patient should participate in weekly orientation sessions designed to acquaint him with the day hospital philosophy, policies, procedures and staff, and to provide a means for determining the most appropriate intervention or treatment.

## TREATMENT MODALITIES AND CONCRETE SERVICES

Following the orientation period, some patients may be seen for individual counseling weekly, biweekly, or monthly, as indicated. Others should be followed mainly through regular contacts with the family member or "significant others."

There are numerous ways in which social work staff can help patients and their families to become acquainted with and to use local support services. This is an essential part of the patient's reintegration into community life. The social workers assist with applications for benefit programs such as SSI, Medicaid, Medicare, disability and private insurance; they interpret laws and regulations and help with correspondence related to any of the public assistance programs. In addition, the social workers should promote cooperation between services within the day hospital and those in the community, and coordinate services already provided by other agencies, such as home health, family service and mental health agencies. Referrals should be made, when appropriate, to other agencies for services such as financial aid, housing, legal aid, placement in nursing homes and other specialized facilities, visiting nurse service, home health aide or house-keeping services, vocational guidance and retraining, senior centers, nutrition programs, driver's training, family and child care agencies. Patients and family members should be appropriately involved in the referral process.

As an integral part of the interdisciplinary treatment team establishing goals and evaluating the progress of each patient, social workers should attend interdisciplinary team meetings when their respective cases are discussed. They should provide the team with a comprehensive view of the patient's perception of himself, his reaction to his illness, his rehabilitation goals, his roles within the family, how he presently manages at home, the family's reaction to the patient's disability adjustment problems, expectations for his rehabilitation, and other areas of concern. Periodic reassessment and care plan review should be performed according to initial goals set by the inter-disciplinary team.

### HOME VISITS

Home visits should be made when appropriate. When made prior to admission, they can provide data for the initial evaluation, especially if family members or "significant others" are unable or unwilling to come to the day hospital. They can familiarize the social worker with the living arrangements of the patient and the community environment in which he must function. This helps identify such obstacles to the rehabilitation process as physical barriers within the home, lack of supportive services, or dysfunctional family relationships. Family or "significant others" can be interviewed and counseled. Finally, patients and family can be provided with purposeful friendly visits as part of an overall social work plan—a service that may be assigned to a social work volunteer.

Upon occasion, the social worker might make a home visit together with the physical therapist or occupational therapist to obtain a multidisciplinary on-site assessment of the home situation.

### DISCHARGE PLANNING

Discharge planning should begin at the time of admission, being modified as the patient progresses through the program. The discharge process is initiated upon recommendation from the clinical team, if or when the patient wishes to withdraw from the day hospital, or when a medical emergency requires transfer to another health facility. The social worker usually meets the patient and his family, individually or jointly, to explore alternatives and to agree on a discharge date and procedure. In some instances, to ease the transition, the patient's attendance schedule is gradually reduced. In other cases, enrollment in alternate community programs is encouraged and pertinent referrals are made prior to, or at time of, discharge. This process is facilitated by having the worker or a volunteer accompany the patient to local community resources, such as nursing homes or other residential facilities, senior center, nutrition programs, and so forth. Conversely, representatives from community agencies may be invited to the day hospital to interview patients prior to transfer.

Two actual illustrations of discharge planning activities follow:

Social workers assisted two patients in improving the hazardous housing conditions that isolated both of them from community life by helping them to apply for subsidies and for apartments in barrier-free buildings. They accompanied the patients to their lease signing and helped with moving and with the related paper work. As a result, one patient was able to be discharged earlier and the other reduced his attendance to one day a week.

A quadriplegic multiple sclerosis patient, after a brief experience as a volunteer tutor for a hospitalized spinal cord injured patient, was advised by her social worker to explore suggested volunteer opportunities in other community programs upon discharge. Follow-up contacts after her discharge confirmed that she had enrolled in a training course and subsequently became a tutor for a local literacy program—one of the services that had been suggested to her.

An example of an innovative program that was initiated for discharged day hospital patients is an Alumni Group that met once a month. Programs were planned reflecting the varied interests of the members, as well as providing intellectual stimulation. Personal interaction flourished in the group, and friendships were made. An atmosphere was created where acceptance of handicaps was fostered and all members were encouraged to share their ideas and experiences. Thus, aphasic and dysphasic former patients could "speak" at meetings and, with the encouragement of their peers, be understood. The Alumni Group enhanced the discharge process, providing a means for obtaining input from former participants in the day hospital program and gathering data for post-discharge follow-up. The greatest obstacle to participation was transportation; many former patients wished to come but had no way of getting to the meetings. Of lasting enjoyment to alumni were special annual events such as picnics, anniversary luncheons, sing-a-longs, etc. Officers were chosen from among the patient group, and necessary guidance and clerical support were provided by volunteer professionals.

In working on discharge planning, a most valuable tool is the community resource file. A major social work activity is the maintenance and consistent updating of the file. Staff can make site visits to various community agencies, services, and programs; their representatives, in return, can be invited to the day hospital. This interaction and cooperation will improve the quality of referral, discharge planning, and the discharge process, creating an easier and more fulfilling transition for the patient when he has attained his day hospital goals.

### STAFFING

The number of social work staff and the depth of service rendered depend on the goals of the program and the available human and financial resources. Essential to quality patient care is a professional social worker as a department head with experience in treating chronically ill, functionally impaired adults and equally experienced in supervision. The department head, in consultation with the program director, should determine what type of social work services are feasible within the given budget and/or staffing component.

Volunteers may be used to assist the regular social work staff. Social workers with graduate training, as well as volunteers from other disciplines, may be available on a volunteer basis in some communities. Volunteer staff members must be trained and supervised by the professional social work staff in order to ensure job satisfaction and program achievement.

Volunteers can assist with clerical functions, such as maintaining the community resource file, and with tasks involved in obtaining concrete services for patients. Patients and families can be assisted in completing applications for public assistance programs, insurance, admissions to other community agencies, and so forth. Volunteers can play a supportive role by escorting patients to visit community programs—such as nutrition centers or multipurpose senior centers—as preparation for discharge. As part of the overall treatment plan, volunteers can assist disabled patients by supervising certain activities outside the day hospital, such as shopping, handling money, eating in a restaurant. They can also be friendly visitors in person or by telephone to patients who live alone. Recording of all patient-related activities of this kind should be made by volunteers and the information shared with the appropriate social worker.

Undergraduate and graduate students in social work will find field work placements within a day hospital an excellent opportunity to gain experience in an interdisciplinary team role and in the field of chronic illness and geriatrics. This work is truly generic in nature— casework, groupwork, and community organization skills are all required. The day hospital will gain much from student placements, but there must be an administrative commitment to the supervisory time required in assuming the responsibility for graduate student training.

JOAN BIRNBAUM

## CHAPTER THIRTEEN

# Fiscal Management
# and Reimbursement

The fiscal management of the day hospital will begin with the initial evaluation of its economic feasibility as a health care option. Once established, the day hospital should be governed by the fiscal policies of the sponsoring institution or organization. Whether it is an autonomous unit or a subdivision of a hospital, its fiscal policies will need to relate to current external requirements from rate review and approval agencies, insurance plans, and consumer groups.

### FEASIBILITY DETERMINATION

In the absence of historical quantitative and experiential data related to the delivery of day hospital services, it will be necessary to use the most comparable data available in order to estimate and forecast operating results of the proposed day hospital program. If the sponsoring institution has an ongoing outpatient department, the process will be facilitated, because its experience would be the logical basis for estimates of expense and income for similar services within the day hospital. Medicare reimbursement of day hospital therapeutic services is achieved under the classification of outpatient services, so units of service will have to be comparable within the same provider setting. For those services that are being offered for the first time, such as recreational therapy, normal accounting procedures for cost-finding and fee-setting can be utilized.

The rate of growth of the patient population is difficult to estimate. It will depend on the availability of comparable services in the community, the scope of services offered, the accessibility of the day hospital to the target population, and the degrees of satisfaction experienced by patients and families as participants in the new program. It is recommended that the forecast of revenues and expenditures be formulated at several different levels of utilization, with conservatism prevailing. (A table of actual utilization patterns experienced during the development of one day hospital appears in Appendix P.)

To arrive at the necessary forecasts of revenues and expenses, it will be necessary to estimate both direct expenses and indirect expenses. A forecast of revenues based on existing reimbursement formulas, assumed volume, and estimated expenses should be supplemented by estimates of income from grants and nonoperating revenue—for example, fundraising, special gifts, and so on. The statement of revenues and expenses should be projected for the aforementioned different utilization levels in order to determine what utilization level needs to be achieved to break even. If certain forms of reimbursement are disproportionately low, this preliminary forecast and analysis may result in further definition of the target population. In a region where the day hospital concept is new, it will also be difficult to forecast third-party payment by private insurance companies. A reasonable approach would be to base such forecasts on whatever fees for service are currently generated on an outpatient basis for each of the treatment modalities included in the service program. Once the feasibility of the day hospital has been determined, even for a given demonstration period, the focus of the fiscal management will be the ongoing assurance of its reimbursement sources.

### FISCAL MANAGEMENT

In order to meet the demands for external review and internal management, it is important that the day hospital develop effective methods of accumulating and communicating the appropriate quantitative data. The management functions of goal-setting, achievement of those goals, and ongoing assurance of their attainment are all important to the successful operation of the day hospital. The quantitative measures that are relevant to making decisions as to what services can be provided, what functions will be performed by which personnel, and how services will be financed are examples of measures that are an integral part of the budget program.

Generally acceptable accounting principles recommended for hospitals should be followed. The specific format of the budget will vary, but it will reflect all income accounts and chart of expense accounts designed to provide a functional and/or departmental record of the day hospital's operating expenses.

The budget design, fiscal accountability procedures, and overall data collection system should be achieved in collaboration with the fiscal officer of the sponsoring institution and any other reimbursement specialist available to the day hospital. The functional record will permit administrative analysis of any significant deviations and implementation of whatever remedial action is indicated. Such measures as length of stay, admission patterns, patient origin patterns, discharge rates, and attendance patterns are important determinants of program planning and staffing. This kind of information will be especially crucial in nontraditional service areas such as patient transportation. What appear to be reasonable rates for transporting patients when considered in contract negotiations may become unreasonable when a quarterly report indicates that patient cancellations that are not reimbursable have increased the cost per trip by 50 percent. Certain special services, such as x-ray, may be available in another part of the institution for the occasional patient requiring that service, but analysis may show that the cost is doubled when costing is done for the aide escort time in transporting the patient to and from the services, plus waiting for him. Accounting procedures and information management in combination with sample time studies described in the chapter on staffing will enable the administrator to pinpoint such areas for special consideration.

The individuals responsible for the various services should be involved in the budget planning and management process. They should be knowledgeable on the most economical ways of rendering quality treatment and will have an investment in making the entire operation a viable option. The overall goal should be systematic accumulation of relevant and reliable financial statistical data that reflect the day hospital's planned objectives in comparison with actual performance.

## REIMBURSEMENT

The current health care system in the United States provides incentives for the utilization of costly acute hospital care and medical services but creates barriers to obtaining comprehensive services for the chronically ill, physically disabled who would like to remain in the community. To be effective, physical and mental health services should be provided to maintain good health and prevent illness as well as to treat those who are already ill. However, although a comprehensive system of appropriate health care requires that the full spectrum of medical, rehabilitative, and psychosocial services be readily accessible, they are not included in the present reimbursement mechanisms. The present sources for possible funding for day hospital and adult day care programs are a fragmented and complicated melange. In the words of Brahna Trager, "This roster of funding sources represents an overwhelming burden in terms of meeting the wide variety of title regulations, grant applications, requirements, the proliferation of paper work, the multiple reporting and claims presentation, placed upon relatively small administrative and professional staffs."[1]

In the day hospital setting, a multidisciplinary team provides an individualized, comprehensive treatment program that includes medical services, therapeutic services including physical, occupational, and speech therapies, medical–social services, and a range of social-supportive services such as meals, transportation, and socialization. The major goal is to integrate these services in such a way that they will meet the patient's assessed needs. The eclectic selectivity on the part of some third-party payers regarding which specific components are reimbursable for what reason induces fragmentation and is a major deterrent to comprehensive quality care. Most fiscal intermediaries classify day hospital treatment as an outpatient service, and the traditional approach is fee-for-service. In a few isolated cases, a progressive fiscal intermediary will recognize and endorse the day hospital concept and set up a basic per diem day hospital rate. This is the practice in some states for Medicaid-approved day hospital or adult day health service programs. Under Medicare–Part B, only certain services are reimbursable and then only under certain specified circumstances. The intermediary will reimburse 80 percent of "allowable charges," and the patient must pay a 20 percent coinsurance fee for total published charges.

Nursing services, nutritional counseling, and social work services are rarely recognized as distinct professional services on a fee-for-service basis in current hospital outpatient procedures and third-party reimbursement schedules. However, if the day hospital is in a rural area, it is possible that the nursing service may qualify for reimbursement under the title of "clinic visit," which is allowable under rural health agency Medicare policies. The same type of visit rendered 10 miles away in a nonrural area will not be reimbursable. Psychiatric social work services are reimbursable under certain circumstances when ordered by and signed for by a physician. Nutritional counseling provided by the area office of aging will be reimbursable within another mechanism. The resulting cash coordination of services is counterproductive in the delivery of adequate care to a needful population.

To further complicate the situation, some third-party payers, such as Medicare, specifically reimburse for services only when those services result in what they consider demonstrable patient "improvement." Interpretations of improvement vary between the fiscal intermediaries, as do their interpretations of other guidelines and definitions of reimbursement legislation. Services resulting in "maintenance" of functional level are not reimbursable, even though this maintenance keeps the respective patient at home and avoids more costly acute hospitalization or delays long-term institutionalization.

At present, multiple sources of funding are usually needed to make day hospital participation financially feasible for a patient. These sources might be a combination of Medicaid and Medicare; Medicare–Part B and self-payment of the required 20 percent coinsurance; Medicare and private insurance; and so on. Some of the sources that currently reimburse for day hospital services are:

1. *Medicaid—Title XIX of the Social Security Act.* This is a state-administered program of medical assistance, with matching federal funds for persons meeting certain eligibility criteria, including income limitations. Benefits vary from state to state, depending on the provisions written into each state's legislation to delineate their proposed use of Medicaid funds. For day hospital costs to be reimbursable, day hospital services must be specifically included in a state's overall health services plan. (New York, New Jersey, California, Massachusetts, and Washington are among the states that have enacted such legislation.) To qualify for reimbursement, a provider must focus its program on active medical and health-related treatment, involving at least physician, nursing, and social work services, not merely on maintenance care. Reimbursement comes under either of the two existing Medicaid service benefits: (a) outpatient hospital services or (b) clinic services. Per diem rates and the acceptability of the provider are determined by the State Medicaid agency or agencies. In those states where day hospital services are not incorporated into the state's Medicaid plan, a sponsor may seek approval by the Department of Health, Education and Welfare for a demonstration project under Section 1115 of the Social

Security Act, which would permit federal matching of the expenditures accrued by the project at the same rate normally allowable under the state program.

2. *Medicare—Title XVIII of the Social Security Act.* This is administered federally, with national regulations and implementation. To obtain reimbursement under Medicare, a patient must be certified under Medicare-Part B; the deductible and copayment charges for Medicare-Part B apply; the provider must be certified by Medicare; and only certain services are reimbursable such as physician visits, physical therapy, occupational therapy, speech and hearing therapy, laboratory and radiological visits. Services classified as maintenance care are not reimbursable, as has already been mentioned. Costs for administration, professional nursing services and social services are reimbursable only as they may be allocated toward providing one of the foregoing covered services.

3. *Social Services—Title XX of the Social Security Act.* Under certain conditions, these funds may be used to reimburse specific day hospital services. Since Title XX is also state-administered and each state has its own priorities for funds allocation, variations will occur from one state to the other. In addition, reimbursable services must be specifically included in the state's overall Title XX Comprehensive Annual Services Program Plan (CASP). Directed primarily toward social services, Title XX includes several day hospital goals such as helping people become or remain self-sufficient, helping families to stay together, and preventing and reducing inappropriate institutional care as much as possible by providing alternative community-based services. Specifically, it includes certain social work evaluation and counseling, recreational activities such as those concerned with reality orientation, nutritional services such as the preparation and serving of food, transportation, educational and training activities.

4. *Model Projects on Aging—Title III of the Older Americans Act.* Possible funding might be obtained under Title III, which provides for transportation and for social, recreational, and educational services not otherwise provided. These funds, awarded for a specified time period, are to be used to support innovative programs that might contribute to overall knowledge.

5. *Nutrition—Title VII of the Older Americans Act.* Reimbursement for hot meals served at least five days per week to participants over the age of 60 might be obtained under Title VII and be

helpful to a specific segment of day hospital patients. Arrangements would be made through area offices on aging.

6. *Certain private health insurance carriers* have reimbursed part or all of day hospital charges; these include Blue Cross, Metropolitan Life Insurance Company, Aetna Life and Casualty Company, Equitable Life Assurance Company, Connecticut General Life Insurance Company, Phoenix Mutual Life Insurance Company, Provident Life Insurance Company, Mutual of Omaha Insurance Company, United States Postal Service Insurance, Champvas (veterans' insurance), the Travelers Insurance Companies, and Allstate Insurance Company. Since this form of health care is relatively new, interpretation to the insurance agent requires careful documentation of the treatment services in order to gain reimbursement approval. It is preferable to have the patient or family complete an "assignment" authorizing insurance payments directly to the day hospital.

7. *Individual self payments* by patients for nonreimbursed services.

8. *Federal grants* given for research demonstrations and evaluations, which permit reimbursement of patient care costs for research purposes.

9. *Revenue sharing funds* in some states and communities.

10. *Funds from various public and private philanthropic agencies.*

11. *Local public funds.*

12. *Retired Senior Volunteer Program (RSVP).* The day hospital might recruit volunteers through this partially federally funded program. Administered through the area office on aging, it is intended to provide meaningful use of time for retired seniors. Needed transportation and a meal for these volunteers can be provided under a local program.

## COST EFFECTIVENESS

The cost effectiveness of health care will be dependent on its availability, accessibility, continuity, quality, and the appropriateness of treatment services. The day hospital helps the individual to achieve and maintain his best level of function. For some patients it prevents acute care hospitalization; for others, it delays long-term institutionalization. However, unless it is part of a continuum of community-based long-term care and support services that ensure its availability, accessibility, and appropriateness, it becomes difficult to prove its cost effectiveness.

Most of the studies of adult day care or adult day health services have attempted to demonstrate its cost-effectiveness as a new health care option in the United States. Unfortunately, the study populations and the units of treatment delivered to those populations have not been comparable. Cost data has been incomplete, and assessed outcomes did not lend themselves to cost analysis. Congressional leaders are seeking solutions to the skyrocketing costs of health care in general and to health care for the chronically physically and mentally disabled in particular. There is an urgent need to develop research demonstrations that will measure the cost benefits and cost effectiveness of day hospitals within a long-term health care system.

*NOTE*

1.    Trager, Brahna, *Working Paper prepared for use by the Special Committee on Aging* (United States Senate, September, 1976).

# CHAPTER FOURTEEN

# Community Relations
# and Public Information

## PROGRAM

The primary goal of the community relations program is to interpret the day hospital to many different audiences, including: potential sources of patient referral; potential sources of private and public funding; potential treatment resources; potential sources of paid and volunteer staff members; professional colleagues and potential day hospital administrators; and legislators, public officials, and policymakers. Many of the same materials and presentation will be appropriate for more than one audience, even though they may be used in different forums, with different emphases, and for different objectives.

One of the greatest challenges in the early stages of developing a day hospital is interpreting the program to potential sources of patient referral in the community. This marketing effort first requires a clear-cut definition of admission criteria, in printed form for wide distribution, with a designated day hospital source—such as the admissions director—where additional information may be obtained and individual referrals discussed. The individual responsible for admissions is a key member of this community effort because the finer interpretations of eligibility and treatment goals are made at this crucial point in the referral process. This initial contact often sets the tone for any future patient/family relationship to the program.

The publication of program information for referral sources can take different forms, depending on the target audience. An attractive printed bookmark outlining bare essentials and encouraging inquiries can be distributed to all community libraries. A question-answer leaflet that tells the family members of potential patients what they need to know is an excellent handout following a talk at a local center or at a service club meeting. A more detailed description of the program objectives, admissions criteria, treatment services, and fees will be needed for publicizing the program among individual physicians, nurses, social workers, and to all health care providers—hospitals, discharge planning units, home health agencies, visiting nurse associations, health maintenance organizations, public health departments, neighborhood health centers, nursing homes, intermediate care facilities, and so forth. Other sources of referral that will need interpretative literature for staff orientation and client use are family service agencies, state and area agencies on aging, local departments of social services, and homemaker agencies.

All informational literature or public communication, regardless of the target population, has patient recruitment potential. For example, a flyer describing volunteer opportunities in the day hospital distributed to church groups, college clubs, service clubs, and other organizations will serve to inform the same audience about the existence and availability of the new community-based health service program. Other tools that are useful for general distribution to the aforementioned groups are reprints of published materials such as feature newspaper stories, magazine articles, and so forth. When more in-depth and/or technical information is requested, the day hospital might offer a literature packet that includes reprints of professional conference papers as well as newspaper article reprints and current handout pamphlets.

Essential to the community relations effort is the development of a speakers bureau service composed of paid and volunteer staff who are skilled public speakers. Volunteer representatives who are enthusiastic supporters of the day hospital concept and verbally skillful can be recruited to address community groups of lay audiences. Staff can be utilized for programs requiring professional knowledge and training. For example, one day hospital was asked to provide a speaker on physical fitness for nursing home residents, and the physical therapist fulfilled this assignment very well. A detailed orientation and information workshop with practice sessions should precede any public appearances by individuals whose capabilities in this area are unknown or untried. All appropriate community organizations and professional facilities should be made aware of the speakers bureau, such as local offices on aging, health departments, home health agencies, hospital discharge planners, nursing homes, mental health centers, low-income and senior citizen housing tenants, nutrition centers, church groups, professional organizations, and service clubs.

A ten-minute slide show or film presenting scenes of the day hospital in action and describing the major program services enables the audience to visualize the program more accurately. It also ensures a consistent, uniform core message. For the speaker, it provides a base of common audience knowledge that should stimulate questions focused on the special interests of that particular audience. Audio-visual presentations can also be used as a self-contained program that can be mailed to distant inquirers, permitting wider dissemination of program information. This has proven to be helpful to communities considering the establishment of a day hospital and in need of concrete program illustrations to educate and orient board members, potential sponsors, and so on, to the overall concept.

The day hospital may receive and/or encourage requests from other health care providers to present a program as part of the provider's in-service education effort. It may be a brief case presentation by several day hospital team members discussing the progress of a patient referred earlier by a local hospital social worker and presented at a staff meeting of that social work department. Or a local chapter of the physical therapy organization might have a program presented by the day hospital physical therapy staff. Small groups of professionals may also be invited to visit the day hospital and to discuss potential referrals or discharges. There are endless opportunities for meaningful presentations to professional and lay audiences. However, to ensure success, certain precautions must be taken:

1.  The presenters must be knowledgeable about the content and skillful in conveying the information. Technical information should be given in a human interest context.
2.  The program content and time limits must be geared to meet the specific interests, level of understanding, and meeting plans of the audience.
3.  Ample time should be allowed for questions and discussion of the material presented.
4.  There must be careful follow-up of individual inquiries and suggestions received from meeting participants.

### EXHIBITS

Health fairs, community programs, senior citizen assemblies, public libraries, and professional conference exhibit areas are all likely locations for a day hospital exhibit. It is well to seek professional advice in designing the exhibit, since there are many factors to be considered; these include the standard size of convention exhibit booths, rental expenses, the cost of transporting exhibit materials, the labor involved in setting them up, and the kind of supervision or staffing needed to respond to questions, hand out informational literature, and so on. If an exhibit can be designed that is self-explanatory, portable by one individual in an automobile, and not too expensive to duplicate, it will receive much more exposure and prove to be very useful. It will also serve as a good background for public speaking occasions.

Another type of exhibit that will serve several purposes is the exhibit of crafts and art work created by patients. Day hospital room and corridor wall areas contribute a permanent exhibit area to acquaint visitors and family members with samples of art therapy, woodwork, and so forth. Such displays provide satisfaction and self-fulfillment to the patient who created the finished product. Authorship should be clearly designated. The community library very often welcomes such exhibits, accompanied by some description and pictures of the day hospital. One library featured the beautiful sculptures made by a severely disabled local teenager while he was a day hospital patient. The occupational therapy staff and community relations representatives had worked with the librarian in setting up the exhibit, which also included paintings, string art, and hammered copper works by other patients.

### NEWSPAPER COVERAGE

Newspaper stories, releases, and photos will be subject to the normal news item criteria: they must be timely, newsworthy, and preferably filled with human interest. Newspaper medical and health editors should be made aware of the program's existence and its news potential. If they are planning a series on nursing home alternatives or new community health programs, for example, the community relations staff person can offer assistance in dovetailing a day hospital story with the other planned material. A feature story on selecting gifts for the physically handicapped could be the stimulus at holiday time. In one community newspaper, a series on volunteerism included a story written by a community relations staff member on day hospital volunteers whose experiences had led to paid employment.

News releases of meetings, public programs, or other events should always include a final paragraph giving essential facts about the day hospital program and indicating how and where to obtain additional information. One of the safeguards that is difficult to ensure in newspaper or magazine coverage is the option of final approval of the copy written by them. Deadlines are always imminent and publication sometimes uncertain, but in the absence of that assurance, an administrative decision must be made as to whether the risk of public misinformation should be taken. An actual example of this occurred when a news reporter did a feature story on the benefits and improved quality of life derived by Medicaid recipients in a newly established day hospital in a rural community. The accompanying photo showed an elderly lady in a wheelchair sitting under a hairdryer in the hospital beauty shop. A very negative reaction ensued from Medical Assistance officials, disapproving taxpayers, and others, whose summary impression was that health care dollars were being misspent. It is possible that an outside organization was supporting the beauty shop service, but that was not made clear in any way. Unfortunately, the damaging image probably remained unchanged despite ensuing administrative efforts to demonstrate the health care focus of that day hospital.

### RADIO AND TELEVISION COVERAGE

Local radio stations are often interested in publicizing new community services. National Health Week, Senior Citizens' Month, Employ the Handicapped Week, and other relevant national calendar designations may be the rationale for an interview with a day hospital representative, at which time information can be transmitted to the listening public. Free public service spot announcements are another medium for conveying the day hospital message.

Television coverage may be less available, but should nevertheless be investigated. One day hospital film was used by a national television network as part of a series on "Alternatives to Institutionalization for the Elderly." An evening news program television crew filming a statewide legislative committee that included day hospital representatives resulted in their requesting an opportunity to film a TV feature program for statewide usage in a series on health care legislation.

### PATIENT INFORMATION BOOKLET

A patient information booklet can be developed for the purpose of interpreting the program and providing guidelines for patients and family members. It serves as a permanent reference for information that has been given verbally covering such subjects as treatment services, transportation, fees, billing and payment procedures, holidays, emergency procedures, and so forth. The patient information booklet also becomes another means of informing the public when it is read by the friends and families of patients, and it is of special interest to visiting professionals who are considering the establishment of a program.

### TOURS AND VISITORS

Since it is one of the newer approaches to noninstitutional rehabilitation and health care, new day hospital programs will attract visitors from other communities and agencies, health professionals, students writing term papers, and foreign visitors. Information-sharing or touring without invasion of patient privacy and staff treatment programs is an important consideration. Decisions must be made concerning how much administrative staff time can be expended for visitors. Some programs set aside one day a month for visitors, while others have found that policy difficult and time-consuming to enforce. An audiovisual presentation or film is most convenient for providing a visual tour instead of a walking tour. Printed handout materials that answer the most commonly asked questions will save a lot of staff time. Fee-charging for in-depth consultation visits is one means of resolving the budgetary consideration of devoting costly staff time to this worthy cause. Fees to cover the costs of duplicated materials is another means of meeting the expense incurred in sharing information.

### DAY HOSPITAL SYMPOSIA

Another approach to providing detailed information about the organization and delivery of day hospital services is sponsoring a day hospital symposium and publicizing it in the appropriate health professional journals and newsletters. A symposium can be structured to include plenary sessions as well as small group observation of patient group treatment sessions. All key treatment staff can be on the faculty and be available to answer individual questions related to their particular disciplines. This encourages group discussion by participants and is educational in the resulting exchange of their ideas and experiences from different settings. Governmental representatives, particularly from regulatory agencies, should be included in the faculty to give up-to-date information to participants on official legislation and policies and to receive feedback on local needs and interests. Such a symposium can be organized on a self-supporting basis by charging appropriate fees. A sample symposium program appears in Appendix S.

### MAILING LIST

The creation of a day hospital mailing list will prove increasingly useful as the facility develops. The names and addresses of all individuals and groups who inquire about the program and facility should be systematically added to an alphabetized list or, if feasible, to a mailing list service. Whenever program innovations occur, changes are made, or seminars held, an established interested audience will already exist for an appropriate mailing.

### COMMUNITY OUTREACH

Community outreach efforts are directed at introducing a new health care package of services to those chronically ill elderly who can benefit from it but may not be aware of the program. Public health nurses should be made aware of the program. Invitations may be sought from local housing officials to present programs in low-income housing projects for the elderly. Senior groups may also be invited to community open house programs at the day hospital as a means of familiarizing them with the availability of services.

A holiday tea might be held in December, or at another time during the year, to honor past and present volunteers and to give visibility to the facility. Invitations should be sent to such potential referral sources as members of the facility's board or advisory committee; any appropriate parent agency staff; supervisory staff from the local agency on aging, senior citizen center, department of social services, health department, home health agencies, social security office, public health nursing association, mental health centers, family service agencies, American Red Cross, senior nutrition centers; church groups; private physicians; appropriate staff from hospitals, nursing homes; representatives from local service clubs; and so forth.

As a public service that also creates an awareness for the community, the day hospital might provide a public seminar or a series of workshops dealing with topics related to the treatment of the chronically ill. For example, an existing day hospital offered a series of workshops for the families of chronically ill patients, which included sessions on an overview of issues concerning the care of the chronically ill in the home and community, on senile dementia, on asthma, bronchitis, and emphysema, on medications, on the changing lifestyle, on assistive equipment, and on the maintaining of financial records during chronic illness.

The day hospital might develop a group of prominent local citizens willing to give talks to patients and staff about their professions or avocations. Such a valuable local resource could serve a dual purpose. Not only would such presentations bring a welcome breath of active outside life to patients, but impressions gained by the visitor and passed on to friends and business associates could prove invaluable for future fund raising and patient/volunteer recruitment.

## STAFFING

The day hospital's community relations program should be the designated responsibility of a single individual, even though that individual may have other administrative duties. Its implementation, however, will require the assistance of many staff members, paid and volunteer, and of other community resources. The administrative objective should be to use every available skill and opportunity to achieve a purposeful dialogue with the community.

# BIBLIOGRAPHY

Aleksandrowicz, J. W., "Certain Specific Aspects of Psychotherapy for Neuroses in a Day Hospital," *Psychotherapie Psychosomatique* (French), Vol. 29, No. 1-4, 1978, pp. 93-96.

Allgulander, S., and K. Holmgren, "Day Medical Care—Five Years Experience from a County Hospital," *Laekartidningen* (Swedish), Vol. 73, No. 40, September 29, 1976, pp. 3339-3340.

Aronson, R. (Maimonides Hospital and Home for the Aged, Montreal, Quebec), "Programs I: The Role of an Occupational Therapist in a Geriatric Day Hospital Setting—Maimonides Day Hospital," *American Journal of Occupational Therapy*, Vol. 30, No. 5, May–June 1976, pp. 290-292.

Austin, N. K., et al., "A Comparative Evaluation of Two Day Hospitals. Goal Attainment Scaling of Behavior Therapy vs. Milieu Therapy," *Journal of Nervous and Mental Disease*, Vol. 163, No. 4, October 1976, pp. 253-262.

Azim, H. F., et al., "Current Utilization of Day Hospitalization," *Canadian Psychiatric Association Journal*, Vol. 23, No. 8, December 1978, pp. 557-566.

Barker, C., "Psychogeriatric Day Patient Assessment--1. Making a Visual Aid Book," *Nursing Times*, Vol. 71, No. 33, August 1975, pp. 1292-1298.

Bendall, M. J., "Changing Work Pattern in a Geriatric Unit and the Effect of a Day Hospital," *Age and Ageing*, Vol. 7, No. 4, 1978, pp. 229-232.

Bergeest, H. G., I. Steinbach, and A. M. Tausch, "Psychic Help for Aged People of Day-Care Centers by Attending Person-Centered Encounter Groups" [author's translation], *Aktuelle Gerontologie* (German), Vol. 7, No. 6, June 1977, pp. 305-313.

Blume, R. M., M. Kalin, and J. Sacks, "A Collaborative Day Treatment Program for Chronic Patients in Adult Homes," *Hospital and Community Psychiatry*, Vol. 30, No. 1, January 1979, pp. 40–42.

Brocklehurst, J. C., "The Day Hospital," *Physiotherapy*, Vol. 62, No. 5, May 1976, pp. 148–150.

Brocklehurst, J. C., *Geriatric Care in Advanced Societies* (Baltimore, Md.: University Park Press, 1975).

Brocklehurst, J. C., *The Geriatric Day Hospital* (London: King Edward's Hospital Fund, 1970).

Browne, C., "Community Psychiatric Nursing: A Psychogeriatric Day Unit," *Nursing Times*, Vol. 72, No. 44, November 1976, pp. 1711–1713.

Burke, A. W., "Physical Disorder among Day Hospital Patients," *British Journal of Psychiatry*, Vol. 133, July 1978, pp. 22–27.

Burke, A. W., "The Social and Psychiatric Problems in Day Hospital Management at Hill End," *International Journal of Social Psychiatry*, Vol. 23, No. 2, Summer 1977, pp. 103–109.

Capelle, P., "Multiple Therapist Groups in a Day-Patient Setting and some Aspects of Group Geography," *South African Medical Journal*, Vol. 50, No. 11, March 13, 1976, pp. 448–452.

Cohen, Margery G., and Stanley B. Cohen, "Rehabilitation and Day Care— Another Alternative," *Maryland State Medical Journal*, Vol. 24, No. 11, November 1975, pp. 71–73.

Congressional Budget Office, *Long-Term Care for the Elderly and Disabled* (Washington, D.C.: U.S. Government Printing Office, February 1977).

Dalgaard, O. Z., "A Day Hospital for the Elderly," *Ugeskrift for Laeger* (Danish), Vol. 140, No. 8, February 1978, pp. 431–434.

Dall, J. L., "Helping Old People to Continue Living at Home. The Contribution of the Day Hospital," *Royal Society of Health Journal*, Vol. 98, No. 1, February 1978, pp. 10–11.

Davidson, S. M., and M. Nicholas, "Day Treatment for the Elderly Mentally Infirm—Letter, *British Medical Journal*, Vol. 1, No. 6067, April 1977, p. 1030.

Davis, J. E., T. W. Lorei, and E. M. Caffey, Jr., "An Evaluation of the Veterans Administration Day Hospital Program," *Hospital and Community Psychiatry*, Vol. 29, No. 5, May 1978, pp. 297–302.

Dawson, M., *Developing a Day Center for Disabled Adults: The Kenny Experience* (Minneapolis, Minn.: The Sister Kenny Institute, 1976).

"Day Care Units for Diabetics," Editorial, *Lancet*, Vol. 2, No. 7978, July 24, 1976, p. 187.

"A Day Hospital for Rehabilitation," *American Journal of Nursing*, Vol. 73, No. 11, November 1973, pp. 1900–1901.

Department of Health, Education, and Welfare, Health Care Financing Administration, Health Standards and Quality Bureau, *Planning for Long-Term Care: An Annotated Bibliography* (Washington, D.C.: U.S. Government Printing Office, 1979-281-202-4043).

De Verbizier, J., et al., "Various Aspects of Daily Life of Psychotics in Partial

Hospitalization (The Condition of Psychotics Presently Treated by Day Care)," *Annales Medico-Psychologiques* (French), Vol. 2, No. 1, June 1976, pp. 154-164.

*Directory of Adult Day Care Centers* (Rockville, Maryland: Health Standards and Quality Bureau, Health Care Financing Administration, Department of Health, Education, and Welfare, September 1977).

Fairclough, F., "Community and Day Hospital Care," *Nursing Mirror*, Vol. 143, No. 6, August 1976, pp. 67-68.

Feldscher, Barry, "Ambulatory Care: The Center of the System. A Walking Version of E.C.F. (Extended Care Facility)," *Hospitals*, March 1, 1975, pp. 75-80.

Fink, E. B., R. Longabaugh, and R. Stout, "The Paradoxical Underutilization of Partial Hospitalization," *International Journal of Social Psychiatry*, Vol. 135, No. 6, June 1978, pp. 713-716.

Frances, A., J. Clarkin, and E. Weldon, "Focal Therapy in the Day Hospital," *Hospital and Community Psychiatry*, Vol. 30, No. 3, March 1979, pp. 195-199.

Frohlich, U. B., "In the Day Care Hospital Instead of in the Nursing Home. Does the Future of Older Patients Belong in Ambulatory After Care Facilities?" *Schwestern Revue* (German), Vol. 16, No. 5, May 1978, p. 12.

Goldstein, S. E., and S. Carlson, "Evolution of an Active Psychogeriatric Day Hospital," *Canadian Medical Association Journal*, Vol. 115, No. 9, November 6, 1976, pp. 874-876.

Guillette, W., et al., "Day Hospitalization as a Cost Effective Alternative to Inpatient Care: A Pilot Study," *Hospital and Community Psychiatry*, Vol. 29, No. 8, August 1978, pp. 525-527.

Gooch, L. A., and D. E. Luxton, "A New Geriatric Day Hospital," *Nursing Mirror*, Vol. 145, No. 3, July 1977, pp. 36-38.

Gurovich, I. Ia., et al., "Place of Day Hospitals in the System of Services for Schizophrenic Patients," *Zhurnal Nevropatologii I Psikhiatrii Imeni S. S. Korsakova* (Russian), Vol. 77, No. 11, 1977, pp. 1726-1731.

Hausmann, H. J., "Experiences with Day Care of Older Citizens in Need of Care," *Zeitschrift fuer Alternsforsch.* (German), Vol. 29, No. 4, 1975, p. 401.

Heinemann, S. H., L. W. Yudin, and F. Perlmutter, "A Follow-up Study of Clients Discharged from a Day Hospital Aftercare Program," *Hospital and Community Psychiatry*, Vol. 26, No. 11, November 1975, pp. 752-754.

Hildick-Smith, M., "Day Hospitals Letter," *British Medical Journal*, Vol. 2, No. 6149, November 18, 1978, p. 1433.

Isdale, I. C., and K. W. Ridings, "A Geriatric Day Hospital: The First Year," *The New Zealand Medical Journal*, March 9, 1977, pp. 177-179.

Isler, Charlotte, "Day Hospitals for the Chronically Ill," *RN Magazine*, April 1974.

Kennedy, Robin, "The Day Hospital as a Rehabilitation Resource," *Rehabilitation*, Vol. 92, January-March 1975, pp. 44-50.

Kiernat, J. M., "Geriatric Day Hospitals: A Golden Opportunity for Therapists," *American Journal of Occupational Therapy*, Vol. 30, No. 5, May–June 1976, pp. 285–289.

Kjørstad, Helge, and Kjell, E. Røkke, "Geriatric Outpatient Facilities. The Geriatric Outpatient Clinic and Day Care Hospital for the Elderly at Aker Hospital," *Tidsskrift for den Norske Laeforening* (Norwegian), Vol. 98, No. 32, November 1978, pp. 1616–1618.

Lamden, R. S., and L. N. Greenstein, "Partnership in Outpatient Day Care," *Hospitals*, Vol. 49, No. 20, October 16, 1975, pp. 87–89.

Laurent, M., and P. Berthaux, "Day Care in Geriatrics: The Geriatric Day Hospital," *Nouvelle Presse Medicale* (French), Vol. 5, No. 37, November 6, 1976, pp. 2475–2476.

Liberman, R. P., et al., "The Credit-Incentive System: Motivating the Participation of Patients in a Day Hospital," *British Journal of Social and Clinical Psychology*, Vol. 16, No. 1, February 1977, pp. 85–94.

*Living Alternatives for the Elderly or Pursuit of Dignity*, Conference Proceedings, Texas State Department of Public Welfare, December 13, 1976.

Lorenze, Edward J., Charlotte M. Hamill, and Robert C. Oliver, "The Day Hospital: An Alternative to Institutional Care," *Journal of the American Geriatrics Society*, Vol. 22, No. 7, 1974, pp. 316–320.

Lurie, Elinore, et al., "On Lok Health Center: A Case Study," *The Geronotologist*, Vol. 16, No. 1, Part 1, February 1976, pp. 39–46.

McNamara, E. M., "Continuing Health Care: Attention Turns to Day Care and Hospice Services," *Hospitals*, Vol. 52, No. 7, April 1978, pp. 79–80, 82–83.

Marston, P. D., "Day Hospitals: A Physiotherapist's View," *Physiotherapy*, Vol. 62, No. 5, May 1976, pp. 151–152.

Martin, Anthony, and Peter H. Millard, "Effect of Size on the Function of Three Day Hospitals: The Case for the Small Hospital," *Journal of the American Geriatrics Society*, Vol. 24, No. 11, November 1976, pp. 506–510.

Martin, Anthony, and Peter H. Millard, "The New Patient Index—A Method of Measuring the Activity in Day Hospitals," *Age and Ageing*, Vol. 4, No. 2, May 1975, pp. 119–122.

Masden, H., "Day Hospital Treatment in a Psychiatric Department in Copenhagen," *Ugeskrift for Laeger* (Danish), Vol. 139, No. 26, June 1977, pp. 1553–1559.

Matlack, David R., "The Case for Geriatric Day Hospitals," *The Geronotologist*, Vol. 15, No. 2, April 1975, pp. 109–113.

Matthes, Mildred L., "Diabetic Day Care," *American Journal of Nursing*, January 1979, pp. 105–106.

Mehta, N. H. and C. M. Mack, "Day Care Services: An Alternative to Institutional Care," *Journal of the American Geriatrics Society*, Vol. 23, No. 6, 1975, pp. 280–283.

Minor, K. and P. Thompson, "Development and Evaluation of a Training Program for Volunteers Working in Day Treatment," *Hospital and Community Psychiatry*, Vol. 26, No. 3, March 1975, pp. 154–156.

Morgan, D., "Gaining Independence at a Geriatric Day Hospital," *Dimensions in Health Service*, Vol. 56, No. 1, January 1979, pp. 23-25.

Morlok, M. A., "Community Resources for the Elderly. Day Therapy Centre: The Role of the Primary Care Nurse," *Canadian Nurse*, Vol. 73, No. 4, April 1977, pp. 50-51.

Nordman, J., "Reflections on the Psychotherapeutic Approach to Patients in the Day Hospital for Epileptics at Creteil," *Annales Medico-Psychologiques* (French), Vol. 2, No. 1, June 1975, pp. 1-30.

Peach, H., and M. S. Pathy, "Evaluation of Patients' Assessment of Day Hospital Care," *British Journal of Preventive and Social Medicine*, Vol. 31, No. 3, September 1977, pp. 209-210.

Peach, H. and M. S. Pathy, "Social Support of Patients Attending a Geriatric Day Hospital," *Journal of Epidemiology and Community Health*, Vol. 32, No. 3, September 1978, pp. 215-218.

Penk, W. E., H. L. Charles, and T. A. Van Hoose, "Comparative Effectiveness of Day Hospital and Inpatient Psychiatric Treatment," *Journal of Consulting and Clinical Psychology*, Vol. 46, No. 1, February 1978, pp. 94-101.

Perez Urrea, M., et al., "The Day Hospital in the Psychiatric Hospital Unit of a General Hospital," *Archivos de Neurobiologia* (Madrid, Spain), Vol. 41, No. 2, March-April 1978, pp. 121-134.

Pfeiffer, E., ed., *Daycare for Older Adults: A Conference Report* (Durham, N.C.: Duke University, 1977).

Pierotte, D. L., "Day Health Care for the Elderly," *Nursing Outlook*, Vol. 25, No. 8, August 1977, pp. 519-523.

Pildes, M. J., et al., "Day Hospital Treatment of Borderline Patients: A Clinical Perspective," *American Journal of Psychiatry*, Vol. 135, No. 5, May 1978, pp. 594-596.

Ridings, K. W., and I. C. Isdale, "The Day Hospital: Efficacy and Cost Effectiveness," *New Zealand Medical Journal*, Vol. 87, No. 606, February 22, 1978, pp. 129-133.

Robins, Edith G., *Report on Day Hospitals in Israel and Great Britain* (Division of Long-Term Care, National Center for Health Services Research, Human Resources Administration, Department of Health, Education, and Welfare, October 15, 1975).

Ross, D. N., "Geriatric Day Hospitals: Counting the Cost Compared with Other Methods of Support," *Age and Ageing*, Vol. 5, No. 3, August 1976, pp. 171-175.

Rubins, J. L., "Five-Year Results of Psychoanalytic Therapy and Day Care for Acute Schizophrenic Patients," *American Journal of Psychoanalysis*, Vol. 36, No. 1, Spring 1976, pp. 3-26.

Sappington, A. A., and M. H. Michaux, "Prognostic Patterns in Self-Report, Relative Report, and Professional Evaluation Measures for Hospitalized and Day-Care Patients," *Journal of Consulting and Clinical Psychology*, Vol. 43, No. 6, December 1975, pp. 904-910.

Skerley, Nada, "Day Care for the Aged," *Newsday*, July 24, 1973, 4,5A.

Slivkin, S. E., "Psychiatric Day Hospital Treatment of Terminally Ill Patients,"

*International Journal of Psychiatry and Medicine*, Vol. 7, No. 2, 1976–1977, pp. 123–131.

Smith, B. K., *Adult Day Care—Extended Family* (Austin, Texas: Hogg Foundation for Mental Health, University of Texas, 1976).

Special Committee on Aging, U.S. Senate, *Adult Day Facilities for Treatment, Health Care and Related Services, A Working Paper* (Washington, D.C.: U.S. Government Printing Office, 1976).

Task Force on the Future of Long Term Care in the United States, National Conference on Social Welfare, *The Future of Long Term Care in the United States: The Report of the Task Force* (Washington, D.C., 1977).

Trager, B., "The Community in Long-Term Care," in *Human Factors in Long-Term Care, Final Report of the Task Force* (Columbus, Ohio: National Conference on Social Welfare, June 1975).

TransCentury Corporation, Final Report, *Adult Day Care in the U.S.—A Comparative Study*, prepared for the National Center for Health Services Research Evaluation under contract No. HRA-106-74-148, June 30, 1975.

Valkonen, I., "A Good Experience in Day Care for the Aged in Tampere," *Sairaanhoitaja* (Finnish), Vol. 22, November 23, 1976, pp. 19–20.

Vance, J. C., "Day-Transfusion Centre for Patients with Thalassaemia Major," *Lancet*, Vol. 1, No. 7913, April 26, 1975, pp. 967–968.

Vannicelli, M., et al., "Comparison of Usual and Experimental Patients in a Psychiatric Day Center," *Journal of Consulting and Clinical Psychology*, Vol. 46, No. 1, February 1978, pp. 87–93.

Vietze, G., et al., "Day-Night Therapy—A Necessary Step towards Better Care for Mental Patients," *Psychiatrie, Neurologie und Medizinische Psychologie* (Leipzig, in English), Vol. 28, No. 5, May 1976, pp. 298–306.

Washburn, S., et al., "A Controlled Comparison of Psychiatric Day Treatment and Inpatient Hospitalization," *Journal of Consulting and Clinical Psychology*, Vol. 44, No. 4, August 1976, pp. 665–675.

Weiler, Philip, and Eloise Rathbone McCuan, *Adult Day Care: A New Direction* (New York: Springer, 1978).

Weissert, W. G., "Adult Day Care Programs in the United States. Current Research Projects and a Survey of 10 Centers," *Public Health Reports*, Vol. 92, No. 1, January–February 1977.

Weissert, W. G., "Costs of Adult Day Care: A Comparison to Nursing Homes," *Inquiry*, Vol. 15, No. 1, March 1978, pp. 10–19.

Weissert, W. G., "Rationales for Public Health Insurance Coverage of Geriatric Day Care: Issues, Options, and Impacts," *Journal of Health, Political Policy and Law*, Vol. 3, No. 4, Winter 1979, pp. 555–567.

Weissert, W. G., "Two Models of Geriatric Day Care: Findings from a Comparative Study," *The Gerontologist*, Vol. 16, No. 5, October 1976, pp. 420–427.

Wilkes, E., A. G. Crowther, and C. W. Greaves, "A Different Kind of Day Hospital—for Patients with Preterminal Cancer and Chronic Disease,"

*British Medical Journal*, Vol. 2, No. 6144, October 14, 1978, pp. 1053-1056.

Williamson, F., "A Day Hospital within the Divisions of a Troubled Community," *International Journal of Social Psychiatry*, Vol. 24, No. 2, Summer 1978, pp. 95-103.

Xander, L., "Possibilities of Representing and Projecting Quantitative Relationships between Inpatient Facilities and Daytime Facilities for Geriatric Care" [author's translation], *Oeffentliche Gesundheitspflege* (German), Vol. 40, No. 1, January 1978, pp. 33-44.

# APPENDIX A / STUDY OF THE NEEDS OF THE ELDERLY

Study of facilities and services for the elderly—from the well elderly to those requiring care at home, in hostels, nursing homes, mental health facilities, extended care hospitals

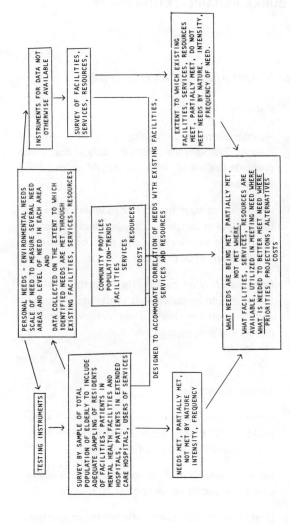

Source: Province of Manitoba Department of Health and Social Development, Division of Research, Planning and Program Development, January 1973, Winnipeg, Manitoba.

# APPENDIX B

## FUNCTIONAL SPACE PROGRAM FOR PROPOSED DAY HOSPITAL AT THE BURKE REHABILITATION CENTER

*Net sq. ft.*

### A. PUBLIC AND ADMINISTRATIVE SPACES

1. *Entrance*

    *Weather-protected unloading space* for 4 vans and 2 autos. The vans load from the side at docks that preclude the use of ramps; autos will unload conventionally.                                              N/A

    *Wheelchair storage* for 75 folded wheelchairs located as close as possible to the van docks. Access to be from the exterior. The area must be secure; no windows are to be provided.                               625

    *Patient and visitor parking* for 12 autos. These spaces should be convenient to the main entrance and designed and sized for use by handicapped drivers and passengers.                                      N/A

    |  | Subtotal | 625 |

2. *Lobby/Reception*

    *Reception and information area:* Provide a semi-enclosed work space for one person. Space for desk, typewriter and two file cabinets.                       100

    *Patient assembly and waiting* space for 15 wheelchairs; conventional seating for 10 people.           600

    *Coatroom* for 120 coats designed for unassisted use by patients.                                           50

    *Security office* located so that it is possible to supervise the wheelchair storage area and the arrival and departure of patients and visitors. Provide desk and phone for van drivers                    100

*Toilets:*

    Male public toilet: 2 stalls, urinal; designed
and equipped for use by handicapped      150

    Female public toilet: 2 stalls; designed and
equipped for use by handicapped      150

                           Subtotal:    1,150

3.   *Admitting*

Contiguous with lobby. Waiting to be accommoda-
ted in the lobby.

*Office—Intake Director:* Space for 3 visitors
(1 wheelchair) and occupant.      150

*Office—Intake Interviewer:* Space for 3 visitors
(wheelchair).      150

*Office—Secretary and clerical:* Space for 2 occu-
pants, 3 file cabinets, supply storage over files.      200

Note: There must be a direct path from the suite
        entrance to the office for people in wheel-
        chairs.

                           Subtotal:      500

4.   *Administration*

Contiguous with lobby. Waiting to be accommoda-
ted in the lobby.

*Offices:*

    Office—Director.      150

    Office—Director.      150

    Office—Secretarial: 2 secretaries, 4 file cab-
    inets.      150

    Office—Clerical, 2 clerk typists @ 150 sq. ft.      300

    Office—Research and planning; 3 @ 100 sq. ft.      300

*Workroom/Supply storage/files:* Tabletop Xerox
machine, shelving for supplies, 8 5-drawer lateral
files.                                                                    150

*Conference room/Departmental reference library:*
To accommodate 8 people.                                   200

                                          Subtotal:        1,400

                              *Subtotal:*                   *3,675*


B.   *PATIENT SERVICES*

1.   *Medical Services*

*Office/Consulting*—Physician.                              120

*Office*—Nurse practitioners; 2 @ 120 sq. ft.              240

*Office*—Assistant administrator for clinical services     150

*Examination room:* To accommodate an examination table, scale, EKG machine, small charting
desk; 2 @ 120 sq. ft.                                        240

*Treatment room/Patient rest area:* 5 beds, cubicle
curtains.                                                             400

*Office*—Nursing service. To accommodate 4 people
single pedestal desks, 1 typewriter on rolling stand,
CPR cart.                                                            250

*Patient toilet/Specimen collection.*                       50

*Clean utility/Medications/Clean supplies:* Provide
"Market Forge" type medication unit; space for
clean linen cart; table top specimen holding refrig-
eration; work counter w/sink, cabinets above and
below; shelving for supply storage.                          120

*Soiled utility room:* Provide flushing rim clinical
sink w/diverter valve; space for soiled linen cart;
space for trash cart; space for soiled supply cart.         80

*Staff work area:* Work space for 4 people; one person in closed cubicle. Shelving for patient charts: 30 linear ft., 2 secretarial desks, 1 standard desk, 3 file cabinets.      350

Subtotal:      1,920

2. *Speech and Hearing*

Located adjacent to the Medical service area.

*Treatment room/Office*—Director.      150

*Treatment room/Office*—Therapists; 2 @ 120 sq. ft.      240

*Group therapy/Diagnosis room:* To accommodate 6 patients in wheelchairs, 2 therapists, 2 student carrels, equipment storage.      300

> Note: Provide one-way viewing window between one therapist's office and the group therapy area.

Subtotal:      690

3. *Social Service*

Patient and family counseling.

*Offices:*

Office—Director.      150

Office—Social workers; 3 @ 150 sq. ft.      450

Subtotal:      600

4. *Conference Center*

Shared by all services.

*Conference room:* To accommodate 18 people, 12 in wheelchairs.      450

*Conference room:* To accommodate 10 people, 6 in wheelchairs; 2 @ 250 sq. ft.      500

*Office:* To accommodate 8 graduate students.     240

*Storage:* Tables and chairs.     50

*Staff toilet.*     50

                 Subtotal:     1,240

5.    *Patient Dining and Large Group Activities*

*Dining room:* To accommodate 55 people, 40 in
wheelchairs; assumes 2 seatings.     1,600

*Table and chair storage:* Access from dining room.     120

*Equipment storage:* Access from dining room.

*Staff dining room:* To accommodate 30 people.     450

*Coffee pantry/Staff lounge:* 5 linear ft. counter
w/sink, cabinets above, drawers below; table seat-
ing for 12 people.     200

*Tray assembly area/Food holding*     500

*Dishwashing.*     300

*Office*—Dietitian.     120

*Janitor closet.*     40

*Toilets:*

     Male patient toilet: Equipped for handicap-
     ped.     50

     Female patient toilet: Equipped for handi-
     capped.     50

                 Subtotal:     3,550

6.    *Occupational Therapy and Patient Activities*

To be located near patient dining room.

*Major activities area:* To accommodate 40 people,
30 in wheelchairs. Equipment to include: floor
loom, 3 typewriters, spray hood, 2 sewing machines,

printing press, kiln and clay storage cart, standing
table, ADL Kitchen for snack preparation.  2,000

*Supply storage:* Open shelves, accessible to
patients for supplies that they are permitted to obtain themselves; secure lockers for controlled supplies.  240

*Patient project storage:* Open shelving accessible
to patients; 100 linear ft. 12" deep, 100 linear ft.
24" deep.  100

*Woodworking shop:* Provide glazed wall between
shop and major activities area for supervision. To
accommodate 8 people. Equipment to include:
1 6' adjustable work bench, 1 6' fixed work bench,
drill press, jig saw, band saw; materials storage
closet; 50 sq. ft. shop space to be enclosed and
acoustically controlled.  550

*Functional occupational therapy:* To accommodate 20 people. Equipment to include 12 suspension
slings, 4 deltoid slings, standing table, 12 side
chairs, work tables. Enclosed, destruction-free
space for individual therapy, 150 sq. ft.; equipment storage room, 100 sq. ft.  1,500

*Patient library/Quiet activities:* To accommodate
a maximum of 10 people; normal occupancy can
be assumed to be 3–4 people.  300

*Game Room:* To accommodate a maximum of
20 people.  600

*ADL Bedroom:* Residential-type twin bed.  200

*ADL Bathroom:* 3 residential types, 1 with
residential tub/shower, 1 with residential stall
shower; 2 institutional types. 3 @ 100 sq. ft., 2 @
150 sq. ft.  600

*Volunteer and staff lounge/Coatroom/Toilet.*  200

*Office*—Director of patient activities.      150

*Staff work area:* Carrels for 3 patients activities
workers.      120

*Office*—Director of Occupational Therapy      150

*Staff work area:* Carrels for 3 occupational therapists.      120

                Subtotal      6,830

7.   *Physical Therapy and Hydrotherapy*

*Exercise gym* to accommodate 10 people. Equipment to include: 1 12′ parallel bar; 2 10′ parallel
bars; 1 hemi bar; practice steps; 1 mat with
cubicle curtain; 2 floor mats 6′ x 8′; NK table;
wall weights; standing table; shoulder wheel; finger ladder; traction unit.      2,000

*Patient toilets:* 2 @ 80 sq. ft.      160

*Group exercise room:* to accommodate 10 people;
2 @ 400 sq. ft.      800

*Physical therapy clinic* to accommodate 2 plinths
and 10 mats. Provide cubicle curtain separation.
Equipment to include: Hydrocolator; hot pack
machine (16 packs); cold pack machine (8 packs);
parafin bath; work counter w/sink; 2 parallel bars.      1,700

*Equipment storage/Workroom.*      200

*Hydrotherapy:* Equipment to include: Hubbard
tank; leg and hip whirlpool; arm whirlpool, domes-
tic washing machine and dryer, linen storage
closet, patient dressing area.      800

*Patient toilet/Shower.*      100

*Office*—Director of physical therapy.      150

*Staff work area:* Carrels for 6 therapists.      240

|  |  | Net sq. ft. |
|---|---|---|
| Staff toilet. | | 50 |
| Janitor closet. | | 40 |
| | Subtotal: | 6,240 |
| | *Subtotal:* | *21,070* |

## C.  MISCELLANEOUS FACILITIES

1.  *Shipping and Receiving*

    Provide only if the BRC receiving area cannot be used.

    *Receiving dock:* Covered, to accommodate 2 vehicles. ... 250

    Subtotal: 250

2.  *Housekeeping*

    *Central storage* for equipment and supplies. ... 150

    *Soiled linen holding:* Provide only if BRC facilities cannot be used. ... 50

    *Trash holding:* Provide only if BRC facilities cannot be used. ... 50

    *Janitor closet.* ... 40

    Subtotal: 290

3.  *Print Shop*

    Equipment to include large Xerox machine w/collator, Gestetner machine, shelving for supply storage. ... 200

    Subtotal: 200

    *Subtotal:* *740*

SUMMARY

A.  Public Spaces and Administration

|   |   |   |
|---|---|---:|
| 1. | Entrance | 625 |
| 2. | Lobby/Reception | 1,150 |
| 3. | Admitting | 500 |
| 4. | Administration | 1,400 |

Subtotal:    3,675

B.  Patient Care Services

|   |   |   |
|---|---|---:|
| 1. | Medical Service | 1,920 |
| 2. | Speech and Hearing | 690 |
| 3. | Social Service | 600 |
| 4. | Conference Center | 1,240 |
| 5. | Patient Dining/Large Group Activities | 3,550 |
| 6. | Patient Activities/Occupational Therapy | 6,830 |
| 7. | Physical Therapy/Hydrotherapy | 6,240 |

Subtotal:    21,070

C.  Miscellaneous Services

|   |   |   |
|---|---|---:|
| 1. | Shipping and Receiving | 250 |
| 2. | Housekeeping | 290 |
| 3. | Print Shop | 200 |

Subtotal:    740

Total net sq. ft.:    25,485

25,485 net sq. ft. x 1.5:1 net-to-gross ratio = 38,228 G.S.F.

25,485 net sq. ft. x 1.6:1 net-to-gross ratio = 40,776 G.S.F.

If the Day Hospital is easily accessible from the Wood Building, the following spaces may be eliminated from the functional space program:

| | Net sq. ft. |
|---|---|
| Tray Assembly Area / Food Holding | 500 |
| Staff Dining | 450 |
| Receiving Dock | 250 |
| Soiled Linen Holding | 50 |
| Trash Holding | 50 |
| Print Shop | 200 |
| *Total:* | *1,500* |

# DAY HOSPITAL

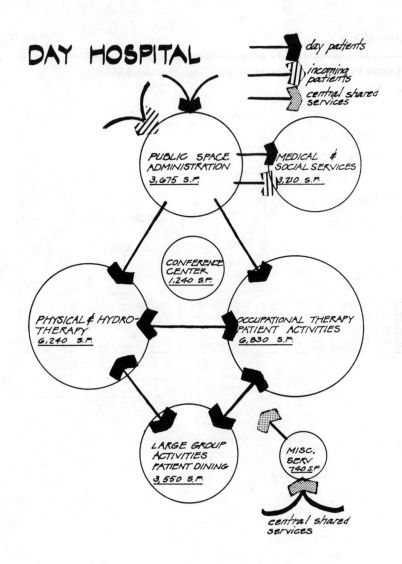

day patients

incoming patients

central shared services

PUBLIC SPACE ADMINISTRATION
3,675 S.F.

MEDICAL & SOCIAL SERVICES
3,210 S.F.

CONFERENCE CENTER
1,240 S.F.

PHYSICAL & HYDRO-THERAPY
6,240 S.F.

OCCUPATIONAL THERAPY PATIENT ACTIVITIES
6,830 S.F.

LARGE GROUP ACTIVITIES PATIENT DINING
3,550 S.F.

MISC. SERV
740 S.F.

central shared services

126

# APPENDIX C

## FLOOR PLAN OF BEXHILL HOSPITAL GERIATRIC UNIT

Total: 13,647 sq. ft.

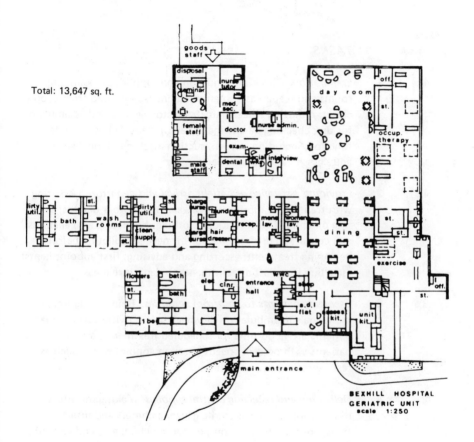

# APPENDIX D

**TIME DISTRIBUTION OF DAY HOSPITAL NURSING ASSISTANT**

(Total hours per week = 35)

*Hours
per week*          *TASKS*

4½      1.     *Preparation:* Checking condition and supplies of examining
                 rooms and rest areas; replenishing linens as needed from supply
                 closet; removing wheelchairs from storage area and assembling
                 for use; checking all emergency equipment daily for proper
                 function, including oxygen, suction machine, defibrillator,
                 and "crash" and "code" carts.

4½      2.     *Providing assistance at patient arrival and departure:* Assisting
                 with transfer to appropriate wheelchair or other devices; assis-
                 ting on and off with outdoor clothing; evaluating arrival status
                 and consulting professional staff if needed; toileting before
                 beginning treatment; escorting and advising; first appointments;
                 escorting from last appointments to departure areas.

3½      3.     *Escorting patients to and from activities:* Reinforcing treat-
                 ment goals in ambulation or wheelchair activities; seeing that
                 patients arrive on time for scheduled treatments; assisting
                 patients with personal needs between appointments, such as
                 rest, refreshments, or toileting.

2       4.     *Delivering and receiving central supplies:* Making inventory
                 of all supplies, such as sterile gauze, catheters and insertion
                 trays, enema kits, solutions, urinals and bedpans, and so forth.
                 Ordering supplies and equipment to ensure adequate availa-
                 bility.

2       5.     *Picking up supplies* at central supply room as directed.

6½    6.  *Assisting with patients' meals and snacks:* Assisting with
          seating in dining area, including wheelchair transfer; distribu-
          ting trays or serving meals, opening food packets, milk cartons,
          and so forth; assisting with feeding patients who require it;
          observing/reporting patients' food intake patterns; assisting
          patients in menu selection and reinforcing dietary teaching.

8      7.  *Aiding with patients' personal care:* Providing baths, showers,
          shampoos as prescribed; foot and nail care; grooming; assisting
          with patient toileting (average three times per day per patient).

3      8.  *Monitoring patients' physiological parameters:* Taking and re-
          cording blood pressure, temperature, weight, pulse, and so
          forth; reporting any deviations to appropriate personnel.

1      9.  *Assisting therapists with patient therapy (occupational,
          physical, speech):* Preparing patient for therapist—transfering
          to treatment table or chair; assisting in treatment practice or
          reinforcement (such as ambulation training, activities of daily
          living, and so on; language reinforcement).

2     10.  *In-service meetings:* Institutional, interdepartmental, and de-
          partmental staff education; attendance at outside meetings;
          individual supervisory conferences; case conferences with
          interdisciplinary team; administrative staff meetings.

# APPENDIX E

## TIME DISTRIBUTION OF DAY HOSPITAL
## ADMINISTRATIVE ASSISTANT IN TRANSPORTATION

(Total hours per week = 37½)

| *Hours per week* | | *TASKS* |
|---|---|---|
| 15 | 1. | *Supervising patients' arrivals/departures:* Assisting with removal of coats; escorting patients to treatment area; recording attendance; monitoring arrival schedule; supervising patients in lobby prior to departure; assisting with outer clothing; monitoring departure schedule. |
| 13 | 2. | *Record-keeping:* Recording attendance, reasons for absence reported by drivers, cancellations, discharges from program, charge slips, receipts, and accident reports from drivers; obtaining and monitoring transportation authorization for Medicaid and other health insurance patients. |
| 4½ | 3. | *Meetings and conferences* with clinical coordinator re transportation problems affecting patient care; with admissions director re scheduling of new patients; staff meetings; supervisory conference. |
| 5 | 4. | *Communications* re scheduling with transportation vendors, families, patients, admissions director, and clinical coordinator; and cancellation in case of inclement weather or other emergencies. |

# APPENDIX F

## STAFFING REQUIREMENTS OF ADULT DAY HEALTH CENTERS IN THE STATE OF CALIFORNIA

Administrative regulations published in June, 1978, for Health Care Services of the California Medical Assistance Program list the following requirements:

54423. Staffing Requirements.

A. The program director, a registered nurse with a public health background, a medical social worker, a program aide, and the activity coordinator will be present during all scheduled hours of operation. Other staff shall be employed in sufficient numbers to provide services as prescribed in the individual plans of care, in accordance with the following minimal requirements:

    1. Centers with a licensed capacity of 40 or less shall provide at least:

        a. One hundred and twelve hours of physical, speech, and occupational therapy per month.

        b. Ten hours of psychiatric or psychological services per month.

        c. Four hours of nutritional services provided by a dietitian per month.

    2. Centers with a licensed capacity of 41 to 60 shall provide at a minimum:

        a. One hundred and eighty hours of physical, speech, and occupational therapy per month.

        b. Sixteen hours of psychiatric and psychological services per month.

        c. Eight hours of nutritional services provided by a dietitian per month.

        d. An additional half-time licensed vocational nurse for each increment of 10 in licensed capacity exceeding 40.

        e. An additional half-time social worker for each increment of 10 in a licensed capacity exceeding 40.

    3. In addition, there shall be program aides in a ratio of one-half for every increment of eight in licensed capacity.

B. Adult day health centers which serve participants whose primary language is other than English shall employ sufficient trained staff to communicate with and facilitate rendering services to such participants. When a substantial number of the participants are in a non–English-speaking group, bilingual staff shall be provided. Bilingual staff shall be persons capable of communicating in English and the preferred language of the participant.

# APPENDIX G

## FLOWCHART OF DAY HOSPITAL ADMISSION PROCESS

A. *INQUIRY-REFERRAL*

Screening interview by admissions director, either by telephone or face-to-face, covering the following points: how the individual heard about the day hospital, reasons for seeking admissions to the day hospital, whether or not the individual has a personal physician, the kind and extent of the individual's medical insurance, whether or not the individual can get to the day hospital.

B. *FORMAL APPLICATION*

1. Patient application: sociodemographic data.

2. Medical information from private physician; previous history, present physical status.

3. Other supporting information: hospital discharge summaries, community agency reports, laboratory data, diagnostic reports, and so on.

C. *PREADMISSION EVALUATION*

1. Interview with client and family by admissions director focused primarily on:
   a. Financial situation and medical insurance coverage.
   b. Can family transport patient or must day hospital arrange transportation.
   c. Explanation of the day hospital program.

2. Interview with nurse primarily focused on:
   a. Patient's and family's goals and assessment of their capacity for adjustment to the illness and the limitations it presents.
   b. Review of health and medical history.
   c. Assessment of patient's functional status.

D. *DISPOSITION*

1. Determination of admissibility by nurse and admissions director. If decision is to admit patient, level of care and frequency of attendance are tentatively established. The decision and tentative plan are discussed with patient and/or family member. Transportation is arranged.

2. Delineation of physical and psychological problems needing further exploration.

3. If inadmissible, referral to appropriate sources of care.

# APPENDIX H

## BURKE DAY HOSPITAL APPLICATION AND ADMISSION FORMS

Burke Day Hospital
785 Mamaroneck Avenue
White Plains, New York  10605

For office use only:
Primary Diagnoses: _____
_____

APPLICATION

NAME: _____ TEL. NO. _____

ADDRESS: _____

BIRTHDATE: _____  BIRTHPLACE: _____
         month/ day/ year

MARITAL STATUS:  S___  M___  W___  D___  SEP___    SEX:  M___  F___

RELIGION:  (optional) _____  NUMBER OF LIVING CHILDREN: _____

USUAL OCCUPATION: _____

EMPLOYMENT STATUS:  Currently employed___ Sick leave___ Retired___ Never employed_____

SOCIAL SECURITY NUMBER:  ___ ___ ___ ___ ___ ___ ___ ___ ___

REFERRAL SOURCE: _____

Address: _____ Tel. No. _____

PERSONS TO BE NOTIFIED IN CASE OF EMERGENCY:

Name: _____ Relationship: _____

Address: _____

Home Tel. _____ Business Tel. _____

Name: _____ Relationship: _____

Address: _____

Home Tel. _____ Business Tel. _____

Medicare # _____ A___ B___   Effective Date: _____

Medicaid # _____ Effective Date: _____
                                         month/ day/ year

Health Insurance policy number(s): _____

Name of company: _____

Address: _____

Contact person: _____ Tel. No. _____

EMPLOYER THROUGH WHICH POLICY WAS TAKEN: _____
        (if applicable)

Address: _____ Tel. No. _____

Name of insured: _____

Burke Day Hospital
785 Mamaroneck Avenue
White Plains, New York  10605

CURRENT AND MOST RECENT HOSPITALIZATIONS

Hospital                    Three most recent                    Reason
                      Dates of Admission/Discharge

1. _____

2. _____

3. _____

Referring physician: _____

Address: _____ Tel. No. _____

Personal physician: _____

Address: _____ Tel. No. _____

Ophthalmologist: _____

Address: _____ Tel. No. _____

Podiatrist: _____

Address: _____ Tel. No. _____

Specialist: _____

Address: _____ Tel. No. _____

Dentist: _____

Address: _____ Tel. No. _____

Pharmacy: _____

Address: _____ Tel. No. _____

OTHER HEALTH AND SOCIAL SERVICES PRESENTLY BEING RECEIVED OR RECEIVED WITHIN PAST YEAR

          Name of agency and person:         Tel.      Frequency/Quantity

Nursing: _____

P.T. _____

O.T. _____

Speech _____

Homemaker Assistance: _____

Counseling: _____

Audiological Evaluation: _____

_____

_____

_____

Name of person completing application      Relationship to patient    Date

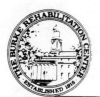

# The Burke Rehabilitation Center

785 Mamaroneck Avenue, White Plains, New York 10605 • (914) 948-0050

*Rehabilitation Hospital*
*Rehabilitation Day Hospital*
*Mental Hygiene Services*
*Bioengineering Services*

Date _____

Name _____

    I authorize any physician, hospital, or other organization or person having any medical records, data, or information concerning my health status to furnish such records, as may be requested by The Burke Day Hospital or its duly authorized representative. A photocopy of this authorization shall be considered as effective and valid as the original.

    I also authorize The Burke Day Hospital to furnish my health records to my personal physician and any agency, which may have need for such information in order to provide health services to me.

Signature _____

Witness _____

Please include copies of the original or reports of the following:

____ EEG                 ____ C.A.T. SCANS

____ EKG                 ____ UROLOGICAL EVALUATIONS

____ X RAY REPORTS     ____ BRAIN SCANS

____ EMG

N.B. This authorization is considered valid for only one year from above date.

Burke Day Hospital
785 Mamaroneck Avenue
White Plains, New York  10605

MEDICAL INFORMATION     Date _____

Applicant's Name _____     Sex: [___] M  [___] F
                  Last        First       Initial

Address _____
            Street        City        State            Zip

DATE OF LAST VISIT _____

PRIMARY DIAGNOSIS (give date) _____

_____

SECONDARY DIAGNOSES (give date)

|     |                  | Historical Information | Present Physical Findings |
|-----|------------------|------------------------|---------------------------|
| 1.  | EENT             | _____        | _____           |
| 2.  | Dermatological   | _____        | _____           |
| 3.  | Respiratory      | _____        | _____           |
| 4.  | Cardiac          | _____        | _____           |
| 5.  | Vascular         | _____        | _____           |
| 6.  | Gastrointestinal | _____        | _____           |
| 7.  | Genito-urinary   | _____        | _____           |
| 8.  | Musculo-skeletal | _____        | _____           |
| 9.  | Neurological     | _____        | _____           |
| 10. | Endocrine        | _____        | _____           |
| 11. | Hematological    | _____        | _____           |
| 12. | Psychiatric      | _____        | _____           |
| 13. | Reproduction     | _____        | _____           |

HOSPITALIZATIONS - INJURIES - OPERATIONS (Begin with most recent)

Date                    Hospital                    Nature of Illness
_____    _____    _____
_____    _____    _____
_____    _____    _____
_____    _____    _____


LABORATORY DATA

The following data must be included in this application.  The findings are limited
to the three-month period preceding the date of this application.

                    Date                              Findings
CBC         _____    _____
Urinalysis  _____    _____
BUN         _____    _____
FBS         _____    _____
VDRL        _____    _____

Please also list any additional pertinent laboratory reports, such as chest X-ray,
ECG, angiogram, brain scan, myelogram.

_____
_____
_____


CURRENT MEDICATIONS    _____

                       _____

CURRENT DIETARY REGIME    _____

                          _____

*138*

Burke Day Hospital
785 Mamaroneck Avenue
White Plains, New York  10605

Name of Applicant _____

Address _____

Telephone _____

FUNCTIONAL STATUS: AMBULATION

Cane [   ]          Wheelchair [   ]

Brace [   ]         Independent [   ]

Crutches [   ]

ACTIVITIES OF DAILY LIVING

|  | Requires Assistance | Independent |
|---|---|---|
| Feeding | [   ] | [   ] |
| Toileting | [   ] | [   ] |
| Dressing | [   ] | [   ] |
| Bathing | [   ] | [   ] |
| Transferring | [   ] | [   ] |

The following services are recommended for the above named applicant to be provided by the Day Hospital of the Burke Rehabilitation Center:

Nursing Supervision [   ]          Counseling [   ]

P.T. [   ]                          Transportation to and from the
                                    Day Hospital via:
O.T. [   ]

Speech [   ]                        Ambulette [   ]

Hearing Evaluation [   ]            Taxi [   ]

Recreation [   ]                    Other [   ]

                                    Other (please specify) _____

                                    _____

Signature of Physician _____     Date _____

Address _____
                    Street            City         State      Zip

Telephone_____

This application is to be returned to the Day Hospital in the accompanying envelope.

## FLOWCHART OF ASSESSMENT PROCESS

I. *MULTIDISCIPLINARY EVALUATION OF FUNCTIONAL STATUS*

    A.    Physical therapy assessment: evaluation of joint range of motion and muscle strength; gait analyses; and prosthetic and orthotic evaluation.

    B.    Occupational therapy assessment: evaluation includes an assessment of patient's ADL status, dexterity, grasp strength, sensation, position in space, stereognosis, perception, and handwriting skills.

    C.    Speech and hearing assessment: evaluation of patient's communication skill; identification of speech/language/voice disorders such as aphasia, apraxia, disarthria; audiometric screening.

    D.    Medical/nursing assessment: complete physical examination; identification of need for skilled nursing procedures; education about disease, diet, medications, home treatments; health counseling.

    E.    Psychosocial assessment, based on interview with patient and family member: personal and family history, social information, educational/occupational information, environmental and financial information.

II. *MULTIDISCIPLINARY TEAM CONFERENCE*

    A.    Patient's problems defined (Problem Oriented Medical Record) with emphasis on functional status.

    B.    Individualized health care plan prepared specifying treatments designed to help patient achieve functional goals. Tentative discharge plans are incorporated.

    C.    Social worker and nursing care coordinator review plan with patient and family member.

III. *HEALTH CARE PLAN REVIEWED BY PHYSICIAN*

    A.    Health care plan is reviewed by the Day Hospital physician and appropriate changes in the plan are made. The physician then certifies that the plan follows the prescribed medical regimen for the patient and writes specific orders.

    B.    The health care plan is sent to the patient's personal physician for his information and review and any suggestions he wishes to make.

IV. *IMPLEMENTATION OF HEALTH CARE PLAN*

    A.    Daily

        1.    Treatments rendered and recorded.

        2.    Assessment of patient's ongoing status with any changes noted.

        3.    Appropriate alterations made in plan to accommodate patient's changing needs.

    B.    Monthly

        1.    Each discipline reviews each patient's care plan, summarizes progress, and indicates any change in the plan.

        2.    Physician reviews and certifies updated plan.

    C.    Quarterly Multidisciplinary Team Conference

        1.    Each discipline re-evaluates the patient's functional status to determine progress made toward achievement of functional goals. Determination is made as to continuation in program, change in level of program, or discharge. Health care plan is updated.

        2.    Evaluation regularly scheduled at the end of three months, but conference can be held at the request of any team member at any time.

## DAY HOSPITAL PREADMISSION INTERVIEW GUIDE

1. Reason for admission to day hospital:

    a. chief complaint

    b. applicant's goal

    c. family's goal

2. Source of referral:

    a. review of primary physician's requests for therapy

    b. review of primary physician's assessment of present health status

3. History of present illness:

    a. onset, progression.

    b. names and dates of previous hospitals, institutions, or agencies utilized by applicant

    c. current medical supervision, interval of visits to local physician or clinic

4. Functional status (present):

    a. ambulatory status:

        1. independent

        2. with standby observation

        3. with minimal assistance of 1

        4. with maximum assistance of 1

        5. with device and 1

        6. with device and 2

        7. wheelchair-dependent

    b. transfer status:

        1. independent

2.  independent with observation

  3.  with assistance of 1

  4.  with assistance of 2

  5.  with device and 1

  6.  with device and 2

c.  eating

  1.  independent

  2.  with assistive devices

  3.  requires preparation of food

  4.  requires feeding

  5.  requires suctioning before, after, or during meal

  6.  swallows solids and liquids

  7.  swallows liquids only

  8.  methods other than oral

d.  awareness of limitations

  1.  is fully aware

  2.  requires cuing for certain activities

  3.  requires cuing all the time

  4.  is unaware but educable

  5.  is unaware and uneducable

5.  Pre-illness life style, occupation

  1.  education

  2.  job history

  3.  age of disability

  4.  age of retirement

  5.  locations lived in

  6.  tobaco use

  7.  alcohol use

  8.  drug use

  9.  travel experience

  10.  marital history

6. Social history

    1. family makeup

    2. additional supports

    3. hobbies

    4. interests

7. Communication

    a. verbal

        1. primary language

        2. speech impediments

        3. comprehension

        4. literacy

        5. style of speech

    b. visual acuity

        1. corrective lens—date

        2. legally blind—date

        3. functionally blind—date

        4. without sight—date

        5. other

    c. audial activity

        1. intact

        2. impaired

        3. with device

        4. date of onset

# APPENDIX K / GUIDELINES FOR MODES OF TRANSPORTATION FOR MEDICAL PURPOSES

The following are examples of medical conditions which enable a patient to utilize the mode of transportation designated. These examples do not comprise an all-inclusive list. Discretion is to be used:

*Public*

1. Skin conditions—unless contagious
2. Allergies
3. Obesity
4. Eye problems (unless severe visual handicap)
5. Upper respiratory conditions
6. Minor orthopedic conditions
7. Mild mental retardation
8. Abdominal symptoms— no incapacitation
9. Cardiac, if no limitation to moderate walking
10. Diabetes, if no limiting visual or cardiac conditions

*Taxi without driver assistance*

1. Fever
2. Contagious disease
3. History of frequent seizures
4. Weakness
5. Orthopedic or arthritic

*Taxi with driver assistance*

1. Mild senility
2. Dizziness
3. Vision or hearing problems requiring escort
4. General weakness and debility
5. Arthritis, moderately disabled
6. Moderate cardiac disability

*Ambulette*

1. Wheelchair-bound (non-collapsible)
2. Advanced senility
3. Hemiplegic
4. Para- or quadriplegic
5. Arthritically disabled
6. Generally debilitated
7. Amputees confined to a wheelchair
8. Unaccompanied children, if warranted

*Ambulance*

Marked or severe cardiac or respiratory condition
2. Head or back injury
3. Fractured hip

145

## DAY HOSPITAL PATIENT TRANSPORTATION MAP

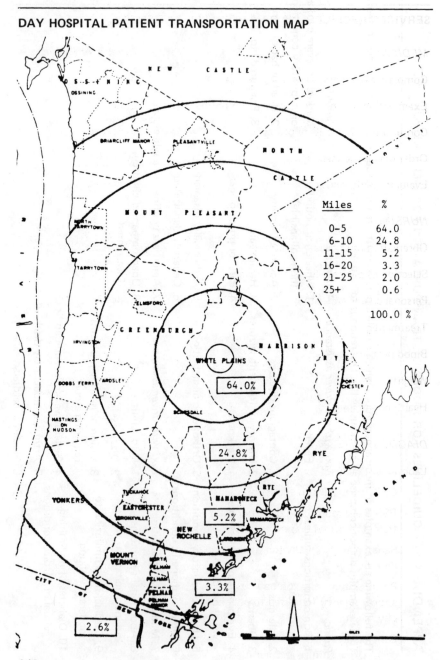

| Miles | % |
|-------|------|
| 0-5 | 64.0 |
| 6-10 | 24.8 |
| 11-15 | 5.2 |
| 16-20 | 3.3 |
| 21-25 | 2.0 |
| 25+ | 0.6 |
| | 100.0 % |

# APPENDIX M

## SERVICES RECEIVED BY DAY HOSPITAL PATIENTS

| *MEDICAL* | *Number of Patients* |
|---|---|
| Complete examination every 4½ months | all |
| Examination for specific signs and symptoms | as needed |
| Consultation with private physician | as needed |
| Order diagnostic tests | as needed |
| Evaluate results and medications | as needed |

| *NURSING* | |
|---|---|
| Observation of signs and symptoms | all |
| Selection of patients to see physician | all |
| Personal care (baths, etc.) | as needed |
| Treatments | as needed |
| Blood pressure, pulse | all: twice/week |
| Weight | all: twice/week |
| Health counseling | as needed |

### *DIAGNOSTIC TESTS*

Laboratory Analyses

| | |
|---|---|
| CBC, urinalysis (on admission) | all |
| FBS every month (on diabetic) (plus fractional urines on unit every week) | |
| Serum Na+, K+, BUN (on patients on diuretics) | |
| Prothrombin times (on patients on anticoagulants) (reported to patient's physician) | |
| Other tests | as needed |
| Urine culture and sensitivity | |

|  |  | *Number of Patients* |
|---|---|---|
| | Chemistries—uric acid | as needed |
| | Fungal culture | |
| EKG | | all |
| Vision | | all |
| Hearing | | all |
| X-ray | | as needed |
| Dental | | as needed |
| Activities of Daily Living | | as needed |

## THERAPIES

| | |
|---|---|
| Physical therapy | as needed |
| Occupational therapy and recreational therapy | all |
| Hydrotherapy | as needed |
| Speech therapy | as needed |

## NUTRITION
(Consultant nutritionist 1 day/week)

| | |
|---|---|
| Discussion of diets with patients | all |
| Discussion of diets with families | as needed |

## SOCIAL SERVICES

| | |
|---|---|
| Group counseling (weekly) | all |
| Individual casework | as needed |
| Family counseling | as needed |
| Referral to community agencies | as needed |
| Discharge planning | all |

## PODIATRY

| | |
|---|---|
| | as needed |

## OPHTHALMOLOGY

| | |
|---|---|
| | as needed |

# APPENDIX N

**DIABETES MELLITUS PROTOCOL**

*POLICY*

It is the responsibility of the day hospital physician and nursing staff to:

1. detect undiagnosed diabetes mellitus and refer the patient with this condition to his physician for treatment;

2. monitor and be aware of the treatment of the patient with known diabetes mellitus;

3. assist the patient with diabetes mellitus to control his condition by teaching him and/or his family about diet, effects of drug therapy, urine testing, and signs and symptoms of hypoglycemia and hyperglycemia.

*PROTOCOL*

I. *Screening procedure for diabetes mellitus*

1. Review records on admission of blood suger tests and urinalysis. If no reports are available, have a random blood sugar and urinalysis performed.

2. If patient has a reported elevated blood sugar in his medical records or an elevated sugar after admission:

   a. Repeat the blood sugar at a random time, that is, two or three hours after a normal breakfast. Record on the lab slip the time that breakfast was eaten and that the blood was drawn along with the food intake at breakfast.

   b. Obtain a urine specimen as close as possible to the time that blood is drawn. Test for presence of sugar and ketones.

   c. Review drug therapy to determine if patient is taking any drugs that potentiate hyperglycemia, such as steroids or thiazide diuretics.

   d. Obtain a urine specimen one and half hours before lunch each week for three weeks. Test for presence of sugar and ketones.

   If the blood sugar is normal and the urine specimen contain neither sugar nor ketones, the patient has random hyperglycemia (latent diabetes mellitus).

If the blood sugar is at or above the following levels, there is a probability that the patient has diabetes mellitus:

|  | Blood sugar | |
| --- | --- | --- |
| | Hours after breakfast | |
| Age | 1 hr. | 2 hrs. |
| Under 50 | 180 mg% | 120 mg% |
| Over 50 | 180 mg% | 135 mg% |

3. If the blood sugar is elevated, notify the patient's community physician. Recommend that a glucose tolerance test be performed to confirm the diagnosis.

II. *Monitoring patients with latent diabetes mellitus*

(These patients have a normal glucose tolerance test when the condition that precipitated the hyperglycemia, for example, pregnancy, infection, steroid therapy, obesity, or other stress, has been resolved.)

Repeat random blood sugar every three months. Community physician may have the test performed and report the results to the day hospital.

III. *Classification of overt diabetes mellitus*
(According to the British Diabetic Association)

1. Chemical (or subclinical or asymptomatic) diabetes mellitus
The patient may or may not have a fasting blood sugar over 130 mg./100 ml. However, his glucose tolerance curve shows a diabetic response. He has neither symptoms nor complications of diabetes mellitus.

2. Clinical diabetes mellitus
The patient's glucose tolerance curve shows a diabetic curve and he has either symptoms or complications of diabetes mellitus.

IV. *Monitoring patients with either chemical or clinical diabetes mellitus*

1. Have patient or family member test the patient's first voided urine specimen for the presence of sugar and ketones every morning for two weeks. Review the record.

If the patient is being treated with insulin or has glycosuria, have patient or family member continue daily urine tests.

If the patient is not taking insulin and all urine tests have been negative for sugar and ketones, have the patient or family member test the urine weekly.

Review the record monthly.

2. Review drug therapy. Observe patient for the side effects of the drugs.

3. Obtain a urine specimen one half-hour before lunch each week. Test for the presence of sugar and ketones. Record on the patient's medical record.

4. Review patient's diet, the prescribed diet, as well as his dietary habits.

5. Weigh patient each month.

6. Fasting blood sugar every three months. Community physician may have the test performed and report the results to the Day Hospital.

## REFERENCES

M. Ellenberg. *Diabetes Mellitus: Theory and Practice.* New York: McGraw-Hill, 1970.

|  | *Upper Limits of Normal Blood Sugar (mg%)* | | |
|---|---|---|---|
| *Age* | *Hours after breakfast* | | |
|  | *1* | *2* | *3* |
| Under 45 | 140 | 110 | |
| 45 to 54 | 150 | 120 | |
| 55 to 64 | 170 | 130 | |
| Over 65 | 180 | 160 | |

Brocklehurst, J. C. *Textbook of Geriatric Medicine and Gerontology.* Edinburgh and London: Churchill Livingstone, 1974, p. 464.

*Blood sugar findings during glucose tolerance test with 50 gm glucose*

|  |  | *Hours after glucose intake* | |
|---|---|---|---|
| *Age* | *Fasting* | *1* | *2* |
| 50 – 69 | 89.7 ± 14 | 162 ± 41 | 98.5 ± 31 |
| 70 + | 99.1 ± 16 | 186 ± 43 | 118.8 ± 44 |

# APPENDIX O

## DAY HOSPITAL PROTOCOLS

### Administration of Medications Policy

*POLICY*

It is the responsibility of the day hospital physician and nursing staff to:

1.  maintain a current list of prescription and over-the-counter drugs taken by the patient;

2.  establish whether the patient is competent in self-medication;

3.  encourage the patient to have his prescriptions filled at a local pharmacy;

4.  encourage the patient to be as independent in administration of medications as his capacities will permit;

5.  develop and follow standing orders for the treatment of common complaints, such as headache, indigestion.

*PROTOCOL*

I.  *On admission*

    1.  Have patient bring in all prescriptions drugs in their original containers.

    2.  Review all medications that patient is taking.

    3.  Record all medications and doses on the Medication Flow Sheet, which is revised when drugs are changed, and review every three months.

    4.  Determine adequacy of patient's knowledge about his medications.

    5.  Test patient's competency for self-medication.

6.   Establish whether patient is competent in self-medication, able to take prepoured medications, or incompetent in self-medication.

II.   *Administration of medications*

1.   Patients who demonstrate their competency in self-medication will take their own medications while at the day hospital.

2.   Patients who demonstrate their ability to take prepoured medications independently will be given labeled unit-dose vials. Family members will fill the vials at home; the patient will bring them to the day hospital and take them without assistance. Liquid drugs are dispensed from the day hospital stock or from a source provided by the patient.

3.   Patients who are incompetent in self-medication will have their drugs administered by the day hospital nurse. The day hospital physician will write orders for the drugs as they were originally prescribed by the patients' personal physicians. The Burke Rehabilitation Center Pharmacy will supply the drug.

4.   If patients forget to bring their medications the dose for that day will be administered by the day hospital nurse. The day hospital physician will write an order for these medications.

5.   When patients present common complaints, such as headache or indigestion, the nurse will administer nonprescription drugs according to standing orders prepared and signed by the day hospital physician.

## Protocol for Disorders of the Urinary Tract

*POLICY*

It is the responsibility of the day hospital physician and nursing staff to:

1. detect urinary tract infections and refer patients to their community physicians for treatment;

2. determine the outcome of treatment for urinary tract infections;

3. monitor patients for recurrent urinary tract infections and the development of renal failure;

4. monitor the bladder and kidney function of patient with neurogenic bladders;

5. recommend urological evaluations for patients with neurogenic bladders.

*PROTOCOL*

I. *Detection of urinary tract infections*

    1. Review records on admissions for evidence of a urinary tract infection.

    If a urinalysis was not performed within the proceeding six months, have a urinalysis performed.

    Method of collection of specimens for urinalysis:

        a. (If no collection device)

        Cleanse the perineum in females or the glans penis in males with soap and water or an antiseptic towelette.

        Collect a midstream portion of urine.

        b. (If patient has an indwelling catheter)

        Clamp the catheter for 30 minutes. Cleanse the rubber proximal to the clamp and aspirate a specimen of urine with sterile 22 gauge needle and syringe from this site, cleansing the catheter puncture site once again following removal of the specimen and needle.

154

c.  (If the patient has an external device)

Remove the device. Collect the specimen as in (a).

Reapply a reusable device or a new Texas catheter.

Send all specimens to the laboratory as soon as possible after collection.

If the urinalysis findings include the following, there is a probability that the patient has a urinary tract infection.

Bacteria 3+ or 4+
WBC  10/HPF
RBC  10/HPF

2.  Have a urine culture and sensitivity test performed. Send reports to the community physician for interpretation and treatment.

3.  Have a urinalysis performed after completion of antimicrobial treatment, or if no treatment has been given, after one month. Send report to the community physician.

4.  Have a urinalysis performed whenever the patient presents symptoms of a urinary tract infection.

II.  *Monitoring at-risk patients for urinary tract infections*

Patients who are prone to develop urinary tract infections are those with:

a.  neurogenic bladders resulting from such conditions as spinal cord lesions, multiple sclerosis, and diabetes mellitus

b.  conditions which obstruct the outflow of urine from the bladder such as prostatism and uterine prolapse

c.  a history of recurrent urinary tract infections or pyelonephritis

d.  an indwelling catheter

1.  Have a urinalysis performed every three months if the patient is asymptomatic. Follow the protocol for detecting a urinary tract infection.

2.  Review records and urinalysis findings for albuminuria and BUN levels. If a BUN was not performed within the six months preceeding admission, have a BUN performed.

3. Repeat the BUN every six months if the level is above the laboratory's normal range. Repeat the BUN yearly if the level is within the laboratory's normal range.

4. Send reports to the community physician for interpretation and treatment. The community physician may have the tests performed and report the results to the Day Hospital.

III. *Monitoring urinary tract function in patients with neurogenic bladders*

1. Obtain urine voiding pattern at day hospital and if possible, at home. Voiding pattern record indicates:
   (a) time interval between voiding,
   (b) amount voided,
   (c) characteristics such as urgency, incontinence, hesitancy in opening and closing the sphincter, and continuous or discontinuous stream.

2. Measure the residual urine under the explicit order of the community physician or urologist.

3. Refer the patient for urological evaluation with his approval and, if the patient requests, of his community physician.

4. Recommend yearly urological evaluations, thorough in content one year, less so on alternate years.

   First year:

   a. Intravenous pyelogram (IVP);

   b. Cystometrogram (CMG)—to measure bladder capacity and bladder wall muscle activity;

   c. Electromyogram (EMG)—to measure sphincter activity.

   The following year:

   a. Kidney, ureter and bladder (KUB) film if IVP has been normal. Otherwise repeat IVP yearly.

**Infectious Diseases**

*POLICY*

It is the responsibility of the day hospital physician and nursing staff to:

1.  detect infectious diseases;

2.  provide treatment for patients with minor infectious diseases or to refer them to their personal physicians for treatment;

3.  prevent cross-contamination among day hospital patients and personnel;

4.  prevent cross-contamination among close associates of the patient by providing information on asepsis;

5.  maintain epidemiologic surveillance of infectious diseases among day hospital patients;

6.  provide information to patients and personnel on infectious disease control.

*PROTOCOL*

I.  *Detection of infectious diseases*

   1.  Observe patients for signs and symptoms of infectious diseases.

   2.  Culture all draining skin lesions.

   3.  Determine probability of communicability, and take measures to prevent spread of infection.

   4.  Assess all patients returning to the program after an absence due to a reported infection, and determine whether the probability of communicability exists.

   5.  Determine reason for the use of antimicrobial drugs.

II. *Prevention of cross-contamination*

   1.  Following recommendations in *Isolation Techniques for Use in Hospital* regarding:

      a.    handling of contaminated materials;

      b.    excluding of patients from attendance at the day hospital during the period of communicability;

      c.    assisting associates of patients at their homes to carry out aseptic measures.

2.    Have Inservice Education programs yearly for the staff.

3.    Provide information on asepsis to the patients in the Health Education classes.

## III. *Surveillance*

1.    Record all reports of infections, such as "cold," "flu," "sore throat," "diarrhea," given by patients who cancel attendance at the day hospital.

2.    Record all reports of symptoms or signs indicating possible infection, such as fever and/or specific signs or symptoms:

      a.    urinary tract: flank pain or tenderness, urgency, frequency of, or burning on urination, nocturia, incontinence;

      b.    respiratory: sore throat, rhinorrhea, cough, sputum production;

      c.    skin: inflammation, pustules, furuncles, draining wounds;

      d.    GI: nausea, vomiting, diarrhea.

3.    Record antibiotic use.

4.    Record all cultures and decisions on treatment.

5.    Summarize records monthly to detect evidence of cross-contamination and other trends.

6.    Review summaries monthly at nursing staff meetings.

## Anticoagulant Therapy Protocol

*POLICY*

When a patient is on anticoagulant therapy, it is the responsibility of the day hospital physician and nursing staff to:

1.   monitor the patient's prothrombin time and report the results to the patient's personal physician if he requests that these determinations be performed at the Burke Rehabilitation Center laboratory;

2.   be alert to signs indicating that the patient has an excessively high level of an anticoagulant drug;

3.   assist the patient on anticoagulant therapy and/or his family in understanding the drug, its interactions with other drugs, signs of an excessively high level of the drug, and so forth.


*PROTOCOL*

I.   *When the personal physician requests that the prothrombin time tests be performed at the Burke Rehabilitation Center*

  1.   Ascertain the amount of the anticoagulant drug that the patient is taking currently.

  2.   Ascertain from the personal physician the therapeutic range for the prothrombin time which he desires.

  3.   Have the prothrombin time tested each week until the drug dose is stabilized and the prothrombin time is within the therapeutic range. Then reduce the frequency of the tests to biweekly or monthly.

  4.   Report prothrombin time results that are outside the therapeutic range to the patient's physician immediately. Send copies of all results to the personal physician.

  5.   Maintain the anticoagulant flow sheet in the patient's medical chart.

**Hypertension Protocol**

It is the responsibility of the Day Hospital physician and nursing staff to:

1. detect undiagnosed hypertension and refer the patient with this condition to his physician for treatment

2. monitor and be aware of the treatment of each patient with hypertension

3. assist the hypertensive patient to control his condition by teaching him and/or his family about diet, good health habits, the side effects of antihypertensive medications and iatrogenic disorders

The difficulty of obtaining a consensus on blood pressure measurements that qualify for the diagnosis of hypertension is recognized. Nevertheless, in order to propose a protocol, dogmatic guidelines will be established.

*PROTOCOL*

I. *Screening procedure for hypertension*

1. Measure the patient's blood pressure while he is at rest on three occasions.

2. Use standard procedure for measuring blood pressure:

    a. Make patient sit down.

    b. Wrap cuff around arm snugly at least 1'' above antecubital fossa.

    c. Fill cuff with air at pressure of at least 220 mm.

    d. Release valve. Note the pressure when the first sound is heard. This is the systolic pressure. Note the pressure when the last sound is heard. This is the diastolic pressure.

    e. Measure blood pressure each time on the same arm.

3. Review patient's drug therapy to determine whether he is taking drugs that raise the blood pressure, such as steroids or adrenergic agents.

4. Classify blood pressure status:

   a. random hypertension: one or two of the three readings are in the hypertensive range (as noted in status b);

   b. hypertension: on all three readings:

      i. Person under age 70:
         Systolic pressure over 170; diastolic pressure over 100.

      ii. Person aged 70 or over:
         Systolic pressure over 200; diastolic pressure over 105;

   c. drug-induced hypertension:
      patient is taking a drug that tends to raise blood pressure, and blood pressure is in the hypertensive range as indicated in b;

   d. normotensive: all three measurements below the hypertensive range.

5. If the screening procedure indicates the probability of hypertension, follow up on these findings according to the classification.

   Status a. Measure blood pressure each week for one month.

   Status b. and c. Notify community physician.

II. *Monitoring patients with hypertension*

1. Review drug therapy every three months. Observe patient for the side effects of the drugs.

2. Evaluate laboratory tests. Community physician may prefer to order the tests and report the results.

   a. Urinalysis for protein every six months.

   b. Serum potassium and sodium—every three months if the patient is taking a diuretic drug.

   c. Serum uric acid—if the symptoms of gout appear.

   d. BUN yearly.

3. EKG yearly.

4. Retinal examination yearly.

5. Measure blood pressure:

   If within normotensive range, every other week.

If blood pressure rises to hypertensive range, evaluate further and notify community physician if indicated.

If the systolic blood pressure falls below 100, repeat measurement with patient in sitting and standing positions on the next three days of attendance. If it remains low or if the patient develops symptoms of low blood pressure, such as dizziness, notify the community physician. If patient is taking vasodilating drugs, such as Vasodilan or Apresoline, measure blood pressure in the sitting and standing positions each time.

6. Weigh patient once a month.

III. *Monitoring blood pressure in patients who are normotensive*

(This includes patients who have random hypertension or have a history of hypertension but are presently normotensive without medications.)

1. If the patient has cardiac disease, measure blood pressure and pulse every other week.

2. If patient has normal cardiac function, measure blood pressure every three months.

3. Weigh patient every three months unless condition warrants more frequent weight measurements.

# APPENDIX P

## PROJECTED SERVICE UTILIZATION
## FOR A DEVELOPING DAY HOSPITAL

(Based on 3 Scheduled Patient Days Per Week)

| Months | 1 | 3 | 5 | 7 | 9 | 11 | 13 | 15 | 17 | 19 |
|---|---|---|---|---|---|---|---|---|---|---|
| Patients Admitted | 7 | 21 | 35 | 49 | 63 | 77 | 91 | 105 | 119 | 133 |
| Patients Discharged | 3 | 9 | 15 | 21 | 27 | 33 | 39 | 45 | 51 | 57 |
| Total Census | 4 | 12 | 20 | 28 | 36 | 44 | 52 | 60 | 68 | 76 |
| Scheduled Patient Days Per Week | 12 | 36 | 60 | 84 | 108 | 132 | 156 | 180 | 204 | 228 |
| Scheduled Patient Days Per Month | 52 | 156 | 260 | 364 | 468 | 572 | 675 | 779 | 883 | 987 |
| Actual Patient Days Per Month* | 45 | 136 | 226 | 317 | 407 | 498 | 587 | 678 | 768 | 859 |
| Actual Number of Patients Per Day** | 2.3 | 6.8 | 11.3 | 15.8 | 20.4 | 24.9 | 29.4 | 33.9 | 38.4 | 42.9 |

*(Based on 87% Attendance Rate)

**(Based on 20 Days Per Month)

(Based on 2.5 Scheduled Days Per Week)

| Months | 1 | 3 | 5 | 7 | 9 | 11 | 13 | 15 | 17 | 19 |
|---|---|---|---|---|---|---|---|---|---|---|
| Patients Admitted | 7 | 21 | 35 | 49 | 63 | 77 | 91 | 105 | 119 | 133 |
| Patients Discharged | 3 | 9 | 15 | 21 | 27 | 33 | 39 | 45 | 51 | 57 |
| Total Census | 4 | 12 | 20 | 28 | 36 | 44 | 52 | 60 | 68 | 76 |
| Scheduled Patient Days Per Week | 10 | 30 | 50 | 70 | 90 | 110 | 130 | 150 | 170 | 190 |
| Scheduled Patient Days Per Month | 43 | 130 | 216 | 303 | 390 | 476 | 563 | 645 | 736 | 823 |
| Actual Patient Days Per Month* | 38 | 113 | 188 | 264 | 339 | 414 | 490 | 561 | 640 | 716 |
| Actual Number of Patients Per Day** | 1.9 | 5.6 | 9.4 | 13.1 | 17.0 | 20.7 | 24.5 | 28.0 | 32.0 | 35.8 |

*(Based on 87% Attendance Rate)

**(Based on 20 Days Per Month)

(Based on 2 Scheduled Patient Days Per Week)

| Months | 1 | 3 | 5 | 7 | 9 | 11 | 13 | 15 | 17 | 19 |
|---|---|---|---|---|---|---|---|---|---|---|
| Patients Admitted | 7 | 21 | 35 | 49 | 63 | 77 | 91 | 105 | 119 | 133 |
| Patients Discharged | 3 | 9 | 15 | 21 | 27 | 33 | 39 | 45 | 51 | 57 |
| Total Census | 4 | 12 | 20 | 28 | 36 | 44 | 52 | 60 | 68 | 76 |
| Scheduled Patient Days Per Week | 8 | 24 | 40 | 56 | 72 | 88 | 104 | 120 | 136 | 152 |
| Scheduled Patient Days Per Month | 35 | 104 | 173 | 242 | 312 | 381 | 450 | 520 | 589 | 658 |
| Actual Patient Days Per Month* | 30 | 90 | 151 | 211 | 271 | 332 | 392 | 452 | 512 | 572 |
| Actual Number of Patients Per Day** | 1.5 | 4.5 | 7.5 | 10.5 | 13.6 | 16.6 | 19.6 | 22.6 | 25.6 | 28.6 |

*(Based on 87% Attendance Rate)

**(Based on 20 Days Per Month)

*165*

# APPENDIX Q

## PATIENT STATISTICS REPORT

1. *FACTS AND FIGURES AS OF MAY 24, 1978*

| | |
|---|---:|
| Current patient census | 128 |
| Average daily attendance | 48 |
| Current average admissions per month | 13 |
| Current average discharges per month | 11 |
| Total admissions between 3/27/73 and 5/24/78 | 726 |

| | | *percentages:* |
|---|---:|---:|
| AGE (Range: 25 to 94 years): | | |
|     Under 65 | 31 | 24 |
|     Between 65 and 75 | 49 | 38 |
|     Over 75 | 48 | 38 |
| SEX: | | |
|     Male | 61 | 48 |
|     Female | 67 | 52 |
| METHOD OF PAYMENT: | | |
|     Medicare/Self-Pay | 81 | 63 |
|     Medicare/Medicaid | 23 | 18 |
|     Straight Medicaid | 15 | 12 |
|     Major Medical | 4 | 3 |
|     Self-Pay | 5 | 4 |
| MARITAL STATUS: | | |
|     Married | 62 | 48 |
|     Widowed | 44 | 34 |
|     Divorced | 9 | 7 |
|     Separated | 2 | 2 |
|     Single | 11 | 9 |
| PRIMARY DIAGNOSTIC CATEGORIES: | | |
|     Cardiovascular/Cerebrovascular | 90 | 70 |

|  | *percentages* | |
|---|---|---|
| Neurological | 25 | 20 |
| Musculoskeletal | 5 | 4 |
| Fractures/Trauma | 8 | 6 |

2. *SAMPLE MONTHLY PATIENT STATISTICS REPORT*

*TO:* _____ MONTH OF: _____OCTOBER 1978_____

FROM:_____ DAY HOSPITAL OPEN 21 DAYS THIS MONTH

PATIENT DISTRIBUTION BY PAY CLASS:

| | |
|---|---|
| Medicare/Self-Pay: | 65 |
| Medicare/Medicaid: | 24 |
| Straight Medicaid: | 12 |
| Major Medical: | 9 |
| Self-Pay: | 2 |
| State Aid: | 1 |
| Total: | 113 |

| | |
|---|---|
| No. of patients as of end of previous month: | 123 |
| Admissions during month: | 15 |
| Discharges during month: | 25 |
| No. of patients as of end of this month: | 113 |
| No. of projected patient days: | 1000 |
| No. of scheduled patient days: | 1011 |
| No. of actual patient days: | 876 |
| Difference from projected days: | −124 |
| Percent attendance: | 87 |
| Average no. of patients scheduled per day: | 48 |
| Average no. of patients attending per day: | 41 |

# APPENDIX R / MONTHLY SERVICES REPORT

State of California—Health and Welfare Agency

Department of Health Services

## MONTHLY SERVICES REPORT

Units: 1=1–15; 2=16–30; 3=31–45; 4=46–60; 5=61+

[ ]  1=Regular  2=Change  3=New  4=Retroactive

Medi-Cal #

Cty.  Aid  Case  F  Per

Name

Last Name  First

Provider #  Project #  M.I.

Date  M M Y Y

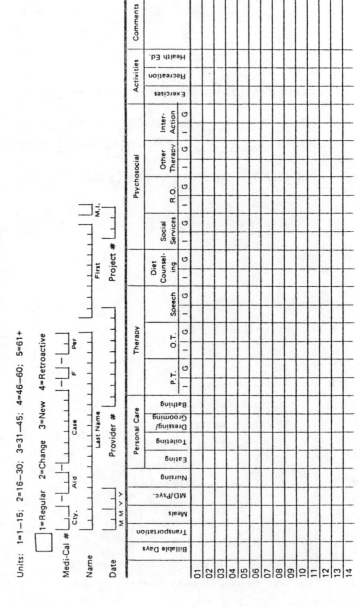

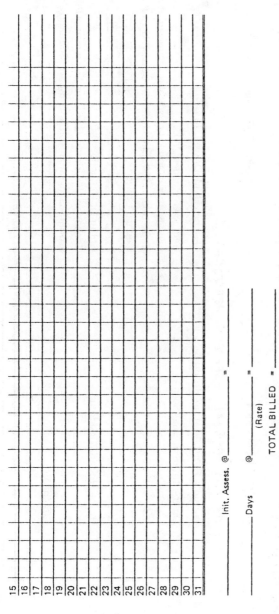

| 15 | | | | | | | | | | | | | | | | | | | | | | | | | | |
| 16 | | | | | | | | | | | | | | | | | | | | | | | | | | |
| 17 | | | | | | | | | | | | | | | | | | | | | | | | | | |
| 18 | | | | | | | | | | | | | | | | | | | | | | | | | | |
| 19 | | | | | | | | | | | | | | | | | | | | | | | | | | |
| 20 | | | | | | | | | | | | | | | | | | | | | | | | | | |
| 21 | | | | | | | | | | | | | | | | | | | | | | | | | | |
| 22 | | | | | | | | | | | | | | | | | | | | | | | | | | |
| 23 | | | | | | | | | | | | | | | | | | | | | | | | | | |
| 24 | | | | | | | | | | | | | | | | | | | | | | | | | | |
| 25 | | | | | | | | | | | | | | | | | | | | | | | | | | |
| 26 | | | | | | | | | | | | | | | | | | | | | | | | | | |
| 27 | | | | | | | | | | | | | | | | | | | | | | | | | | |
| 28 | | | | | | | | | | | | | | | | | | | | | | | | | | |
| 29 | | | | | | | | | | | | | | | | | | | | | | | | | | |
| 30 | | | | | | | | | | | | | | | | | | | | | | | | | | |
| 31 | | | | | | | | | | | | | | | | | | | | | | | | | | |

_____ Init. Assess. @ _____ = _____

_____ Days @ _____ = _____
                (Rate)

TOTAL BILLED = _____

This is to certify that the BILLING information is true and accurate and complete. The reimbursement to be received does not exceed the usual and customary charges made to the general public. I understand that payment and satisfaction of this claim will be from Federal and State funds. In addition, I certify that I will seek payment from the patient for the amount shown on the Medi-Cal ID card as the patient's share of cost (liability), and I will neither claim nor accept payment from the Medi-Cal program for that amount. I understand that any false claims, statements or documents, or concealment of a material fact, may be prosecuted under applicable State or Federal laws.

Signature and Title of Provider Representative          White Copy – ADHC Unit; Green Copy – Provider          Date

IMS 1023 (8/78)

# APPENDIX S / PROGRAM: SYMPOSIUM ON THE DAY HOSPITAL IN THE HEALTH CARE DELIVERY SYSTEM

Presiding: Fletcher H. McDowell, M.D., Medical Director, The Burke Rehabilitation Center
Winifred Masterson Burke Professor of Rehabilitation Medicine,
Cornell University Medical College

## PLENARY SESSION
Wednesday, May 21, 1975

9:30 A.M. OPENING REMARKS Alfred B. DelBello, Westchester County Executive

*THE DAY HOSPITAL: A SERIES OF PERSPECTIVES*

9:45 A.M. Within a Rehabilitation Hospital Fletcher H. McDowell, M.D.

10:00 A.M. On the International Scene George G. Reader, M.D.
Livingston Farrand Professor and Chairman of the
Department of Public Health at Cornell University
Medical College

Intermission

11:00 A.M. In the United Kingdom Robin D. Kennedy, M.D.
Consultant Physician, Geriatric Assessment Unit,
Stobhill General Hospital, Glasgow, Scotland

12:00 Noon Luncheon

*THE BURKE DAY HOSPITAL EXPERIENCE—PART ONE*

1:00 P.M. Charlotte M. Hamill, M.A., M.S.S.W Co-Directors, Burke Day Hospital
Robert C. Oliver, M.A.
Lee Gurel, PhD., Day Hospital Research Consultant

*CONCURRENT WORKSHOPS AND DEMONSTRATIONS BY DAY HOSPITAL STAFF*

2:00 P.M.

Physical Therapy Program and Staffing — Renee Schlesinger, R.P.T., Director, Physical Therapy

Occupational Therapy Program and Staffing — Rosemarie Williams, O.T.R., Director, Occupational Therapy

Patient Activities Program — Priscilla Adams, B.A., Director, Patient Activities

Speech and Hearing — Joyce D. Vitale, M.A., Director, Speech Pathology

3:00 P.M.

Nutritional Counseling and Patient Diet Program — Juliana Snyder, B.S., Director, Nutrition Planning

Nursing Services — Maureen Saouter, R.N., B.S.N., M.S., Assistant Administrator for Clinical Services, Day Hospital

Social–Psychological Services — Raesa Kaiteris, M.S.S.W., Director, Social Services

Medicaid Reimbursement — J. Melvin Merchant, DHEW, Office of Program Innovation, Medical Services Administration

Faculty and Registrants

4:30 P.M.

Cocktail Hour—Burke House

PLENARY SESSION
Thursday, May 22, 1975

9:30 A.M.

*THE BURKE DAY HOSPITAL EXPERIENCE–PART TWO: FINDINGS TO DATE*

Robert C. Oliver, M.A.
Charlotte M. Hamill, M.A., M.S.S.W.
Mary Ann Lewis, PhD., Research Associate, The Day Hospital
Neville Dougherty, PhD.
Lee Gurel, PhD.     Day Hospital Research Consultants
John F. Walsh, PhD.

Intermission

| 10:45 A.M. | *THE PHYSICIAN'S ROLE IN THE DAY HOSPITAL* | |
| | Chairman: Stuart S. Blauner, M.D. | Physician-in-Charge, Cardiopulmonary Services, The Burke Rehabilitation Center |
| | Robert E. Lee, M.D. | Internist and Referring Physician |
| | Mary Lou Bourque, R.N. | Certified Nurse Practitioner, The Day Hospital |
| | Joel S. Feigenson, M.D. | Attending Physician, Neurology, The Burke Rehabilitation Center |
| | Peter H. Stern, M.D. | Physician-in-Charge, Physical Medicine and Rehabilitation, The Burke Rehabilitation Center |
| 12:00 Noon | Luncheon | |
| | *CONCURRENT WORKSHOPS AND DEMONSTRATIONS BY DAY HOSPITAL STAFF* | |
| 1:15 – 2:15 P.M. | Problem-Oriented Medical Records | Maureen Saouter |
| | Facility Planning and Equipment | Charlotte M. Hamill |
| | | Priscilla Adams |
| | Interpreting a New Service to the Community | Helen Proctor, B.A., Public Information Director, The Day Hospital |
| | | Elizabeth Lincoln, B.A., Public Relations Consultant |
| | Medicaid Reimbursement | J. Melvin Merchant |
| 2:30 – 3:30 P.M. | Architectural Consultation to Patients at Home | R. Marcantonio, R.A., A.I.A. |
| | | Apkar Omartian, R.A., A.I.A. |
| | Role of the Volunteer in The Day Hospital | Priscilla Adams |
| | | Emily Beard, Day Hospital Volunteer |
| | Medicaid Reimbursement | J. Melvin Merchant |

# INDEX